Emmanuelle Galland

Feeding Success:

A Nutrition Blueprint to Fuel Busy Professionals and Business Travelers

Disclaimer: Emmanuelle Galland is not a medical doctor, and nothing in this book is intended to diagnose, treat or cure any medical condition, illness or disease. The content of this book is for general instruction only. Each person's physical, emotional, and spiritual condition is unique. If you have a medical concern, consult a physician.

For information, contact Emmanuelle Galland at www.zenberrymix.com and www.gojifitness.com

Published by Goji Fitness LLC
New York

Cover and Interior Design by Kristen Best

Printed in the United States of America

ISBN-10: 0990680401
ISBN-13: 978-0-9906804-0-6

DEDICATION

For my parents
Martine and Philippe

Feeding Success

TABLE OF CONTENTS

	Acknowledgements	ix
	PART I: GOAL PLANNING	1
1	Set Your Goals	2
2	Change Your Brain and Your Belief System	14
3	Self-Assess the State of Your Health	29
4	The Five Principles of Goal-Directed Nutrition	37
	1. Food is Information	42
	2. Food is Energy	47
	3. What You Eat, Digest and Don't Excrete	58
	4. Nutrition Beyond Food	63
	5. A Bio-Individual Blueprint	66
	PART II: GOAL-DIRECTED NUTRITION	72
5	Milestone 1: Eat For Energy and Attractiveness	73
6	Milestone 2: Sleep for Clarity and Youthfulness	139
7	Milestone 3: Exercise for Strength and Longevity	156
8	Milestone 4: Team Up for Support and Connection	177
9	Milestone 5: Slow Down to Focus and Innovate	190

PART III: CALLING YOU INTO ACTION 201

Appendix 1: On-The-Go Snacks 204

Appendix 2: Feeding Success Superfoods Trail Mix 205

Appendix 3: Feeding Success 4-Day Menu Sample 1 (Late Summer) 206

Appendix 4: Feeding Success 4-Day Menu Sample 2 (On The Road) 207

Appendix 5: Feeding Success Power Breakfasts 208

Appendix 6: Dining-Out Questionnaire 209

Appendix 7: Sample On-The-Go Workout Schedule 210

ACKNOWLEDGEMENT

Special thanks to Shane Moran for his continuous support throughout the development of this book, and to Joshua Rosenthal for inspiring me to dream big and giving me the tools to pursue my calling to help people take charge of their health.

Feeding Success

PART I
GOAL PLANNING

1.
SET YOUR GOALS

CONGRATULATIONS! By picking up this book, you've embarked on a journey that will change your relationship with food and what nurtures you for good. You'll learn a new way to eat and take care of yourself. You'll experience an abundance of energy, self-confidence, ease and clarity in the way you think and feel as a result. You'll find yourself more attractive and powerful in your own skin, and able to dare greatly, taking your career and your life to the next level. And you'll gradually see any aches and pains you may have disappear as you step out of your own way and let your body self-regulate and heal.

As a holistic health, fitness and nutrition coach certified by the Institute for Integrative Nutrition (IIN), the American Association of Drugless Practitioners (AADP) and the National Academy of Sports Medicine (NASM), I'm here to introduce you to a new way of eating and taking care of yourself that I have developed over a decade of weekly travel as a management consultant and in my coaching.

The Feeding Success Nutrition Blueprint is based on goal-directed nutrition (GDN), an integrative approach to health and nutrition for the busy professional and frequent business traveler. It is an experience made up of simple steps, which will tap into your intuition and intelligence, inspiring you to create new habits that elevate you through your personal glass ceiling without burning out.

The world needs you to shine brightly, to benefit from your talent, to hear your voice and implement your ideas. Your employer is providing you with the platform to shine with access to infrastructure, manpower and clients. GDN will provide you with a nutrition blueprint to feel your best so you can seize opportunities. Health is a vehicle to help you reach your life's destination. There is no greater high than realizing your fullest career potential and being vibrantly healthy to enjoy your success with the people you love.

Do you remember when you graduated from college how eager you were to make a difference in the world? Your head was bursting with ideas and your body was burning with the desire to power the realization of each and every one of them. You were creative, audacious, and courting the best companies in the world with your unique talent.

I was right there with you. At the end of my last year of college in Sweden, looking for a job and running out of money to stay abroad, I sent an email to the leader of PwC Management Consulting in Malmö. I included my résumé and, not feeling the least pretentious, requested an interview to share my ideas with him: "I think PwC should build a national project management consulting practice that uses some of my ideas to motivate and build competence within teams to increase the success rate of its projects!"

I showed up to the meeting with that fearless confidence only a young, inexperienced person possesses. I presented my model using transparent slides on an overhead projector, speaking half in broken Swedish and half in English. I felt so excited, inspired and eager to create something beautiful and unique for this prestigious global firm. The presentation impressed enough that I was flown to Stockholm to meet with partners the next day and was hired for my dream job, assisting a PwC director to build a new project management practice nationally.

Fast-forward to age 30. After years of stress, my health brought me to my knees and I had to take two months' medical leave of absence to begin to heal. I was diagnosed with an auto-immune disorder called Graves' disease, and was suffering from insomnia, thyroid disorder, adrenal exhaustion, arrhythmia (a condition where the heart beats abnormally), drastic weight loss, eye and digestion issues, anxiety and memory loss. My resting heart rate was 120 bpm and walking reached 200 bpm. I could not walk. I felt emotionally drained and too tired to think or feel passionate about anything. Flying made me sick, which conflicted with the 100% travel expectation to perform my job. My stress threshold was lower than low. It was the classic burnout scenario and I had no idea how to fix myself to prevent myself burning out again.

Conventional medicine presented me with three options to heal: pills, radioactive iodine or surgery. All these were focused on a single symptom of my stress-induced condition: a hyperactive thyroid. But my physicians did not have a comprehensive roadmap to help me understand and treat the root cause of Graves' disease, burnout or other digestive and memory loss issues.

There is a place for modern medicine, especially in emergency situations. I feared a heart attack, so alongside some necessary bed-rest, I opted for the beta-blocker pills for a few weeks to control the arrhythmia and I took anti-thyroid drugs to control the production of my thyroid hormones to help calm my heart down immediately. I also worked relentlessly to create my own 'blueprint to recovery' and naturally control my auto-immune condition to get off medication as fast as I could. I succeeded in healing all my health issues. It took me three years to get it right, to learn and experiment with foods and lifestyle changes, to consult with Traditional Chinese Medicine (TCM) herbalists, acupuncturists, Ayurvedic physicians and open-minded Western physicians, and learn what I needed to know from nutritional therapy to chemically balance my body. I restored my immune and digestive systems, balanced my hormones and my thyroid, strengthened my adrenal glands, cured my insomnia, increased my energy levels and calmed my auto-immune markers. I gained a deep understanding of my body's needs and triggers for health and disease.

Inspired to help others, I invested further in my parallel career in the field of health, fitness and nutrition, which had started in college in France and continued after I moved to the US from Sweden. I operated this as a hobby on the side of my job in Corporate America, but decided to return to school at the Institute for Integrative Nutrition for more education. Soon, my career was rocketing in my corporate job as my health grew stronger. I had more energy, my productivity increased and I earned back two hours a day of me-time to dedicate to my hobby. I gave wellness talks, organized wellness challenges both small and substantial, and helped hundreds of individuals reclaim their health and thrive in their career, avoiding burning out.

Today, I am here to share that very roadmap with you.

My intention with goal-directed nutrition is to help you take better care of yourself, to reach your goals, to preserve your creative and intelligent brain, to protect your liveliness and youth, and to teach you how to control the fire in your belly so that it does not spread or burn your tissues and organs. (Think heart attack, mental health issues, arthritis, swelling, skin issues, all emanating from underlying inflammation, which is essentially excess heat). Studying the 5,000-year-old Indian system of medicine Ayurveda, I learned that the fire energy is what helps us to build the career of our dreams (or family, home, retirement savings, anything) in our 20s and 30s, but too much fire will literally burn us out.

Thriving in Corporate America and surviving business travel depends on mastering the five steps of goal-directed nutrition (the 5 GDN Milestones you'll come across in Part II). There is no one diet or lifestyle to fit all. How you'll reach your goals and implement the five steps will vary based on your bio-individuality, your unique circumstances and your personal intentions. GDN will help you zero in on what works best for you in order to reach your career goals instead of sacrificing your health and life in their pursuit.

The biggest hindrance to realizing your potential is not a lack of opportunities, but poor health. Despite a rise in corporate wellness programs, more and more people are exhausted and burning out before their career goes anywhere, or when they have reached the higher ranks of the company finding themselves unable to enjoy their hard-earned status, taking leave of absence, suffering from heart disease, diabetes, obesity, and cancer, sometimes fatally. Diagnosis of anxiety and depression, sleep disorders, infertility, digestive disorders, auto-immune disease, and so on are at an all-time high. Rising healthcare costs in America, companies' largest expense, are linked predominantly to heart disease and cancer. Even our politicians have named the state of America's health as the greatest threat to our competitiveness.

With goal-directed nutrition, you will be your own guide in supporting yourself back to top health and learning how to integrate your new diet and lifestyle into your career roadmap, step by step. Soon you'll be saying: "I didn't know how bad I felt until I knew what it felt like to feel good".

There are three ways to read this book:

1. The essential read, centered around the instructional content, i.e. the dietary and lifestyle "prescriptions" which will instruct you on the steps to better your health.

2. The workbook, which is made up of questions and a self-assessment (the GDN Circle of Health) to help you reflect upon your current way of thinking and doing things. You already have many of the answers inside of you about how to fix your own issues. Through questioning, it is my intention to reveal them. If you're serious about becoming more successful in your life, I highly recommend you answer the questions as you read through. This is where the transformative process begins.

3. Emma's Story is an optional read to provide some illustration to the essential read and the workbook. It describes my personal experience building my own dietary guidelines and lifestyle.

SET YOUR GOALS

The first step in goal-directed nutrition is to Set Your Goals. Take a couple of minutes now to get in touch with what you want and why you want it. First, close your eyes, take a deep breath, and envision the future...

Open your eyes.

Be as specific as you possibly can when answering the questions below and make sure you dream big. Minimizing your goals will not motivate you as much as shooting for what you truly deeply want in your life, even if you have no idea how to get there. Trust the process! When you feel your best, you will know it.

Feeding Success appealed to me because I want to achieve...

A Healthy rebalanced autoimmune system, a balanced and joyful life, that includes time for friends, spectacles, travel and work + creative work.

I want to achieve these goals because I am currently limited in…

all of the above HEALTH, LIFESTYLE, WORK

When I have reached my goals, my life will be different in that…
(Describe your vision for your life.)

I will not live at ar for work.
I will be more effective
I will work efficiently in less time
I will be more focused
Exercise will be incorporated
into each day & meditation
and sharing myself more freely

When I have achieved my goals, new doors will open for me,
like… *(Describe the opportunities you can expect.)*

I will no longer push everything
to my limit
I will stand more erect &
be relaxed
I will shine from optimism,
passion & sincerity

And every day I will feel… *(Describe your desired mood and feelings.)*

more energetic, focused
less suspicious, guarded
Open hearted
an "increased sense of purpose,
connectedness & belonging."

HONOR THE ATHLETE WITHIN

Important decisions and actions should stem from absolute mental clarity, emotional stability and physical precision. Think about the professional athlete for a minute. It makes sense that the athlete would seek nutrition counseling to improve performance, invest in his sleep and body work for recovery, and practice breathing, relaxation and meditation to focus his mind as he prepares for a big game, right?

Well, to the business professional, isn't choosing a job, preparing a sales pitch, and presenting a new idea to leadership the same as scoring a winning goal to the athlete? You are the super-athlete of Corporate America. And if you are a consultant, you are traveling just as much as the pro athlete is too!

Yet many business professionals like you and me never find the time for self-care, fitness and nutrition to perform at our best. Why on earth would we have to pull an all-nighter to finish a PowerPoint presentation for a client meeting the next day, if we had all this time at our disposal?

I've wondered about that a lot. I suspect there's a perception that the mind functions independently from the body. Do you think the athlete only needs to tend to his physique and not his mind? In fact, anyone who knows anything about sports will tell you that the great athlete presents a perfect synergy. He proves to us that a healthy body nurtures a sharper and quicker brain power, as well as good emotional instincts and intuition.

Even though you're sitting behind a desk and not out on the field, every corporate professional should start thinking with the same mindset as the athlete. To think clearly, the body needs to be in prime condition. To get a good gut feeling, your digestive system needs to be strong. If you're suffering from a protruding belly, bloating, gas, and constipation, your gut instinct can be severely impaired. You could be a much faster intuitive thinker with a healthy gut.

Sadly, instead of caring for ourselves proactively, we reach out to doctors when the disease has already stricken, sometimes too late to heal. Sickness does not happen overnight. It takes decades to develop. Cancer for instance, depending on the kind, can take decades to manifest as the vast majority of malignancies aren't palpable and don't create symptoms for several years, sometimes decades. The choices you make today will determine your fate tomorrow, and 20, 30, even 50 years from now. According to the American Cancer Society, "About half of all men and one third of all women in the US will develop cancer during their lifetimes." It is time to reveal the athlete within and change your mindset to thrive.

Goal-directed nutrition will balance and further your mental, emotional and physical aptitudes. Living inside a vibrantly healthy body will enable you to:

- Develop your intellectual abilities, think more clearly and creatively, and better innovate;

- Protect your mind against dementia, depression, and anxiety, and reduce the risk of Alzheimer's disease;

- Conserve your physical youth, become more attractive, and have abundant energy levels;

- Maintain a healthy weight throughout your life, prevent chronic fatigue and increased risk of cancer, heart disease, auto-immune disorders, and other ailments plaguing Corporate America;

- Increase your sense of purpose, connectedness and belonging, which is all the more challenging in today's fast-paced, virtual and oddly estranged business world;

- Develop nurturing relationships and tap into your emotional intelligence.

EMMA'S STORY

I remember the exact time I first broke through my personal glass ceiling. How scary! But what a high at the same time!

I was working as a manager for PwC in New York and had just arrived in Florida to attend a three-day privacy and security conference with my boss and co-workers. Unexpectedly, my boss, a renowned industry leader and speaker at the event, asked me to fly out to Maine in his place the next day to pitch a proposal as the lead presenter in front of a new client's executive leadership.

I was terrified! I had never done anything like this before. I was not prepared, nor anywhere near as savvy, knowledgeable and eloquent as my boss to be able to improvise. I spoke with a French accent. And the client stakeholders were expecting him, not me. Not only that. Our company's partner, whom I had never met, was also uncertain about this last-minute switch.

As the story goes, this particular meeting ended up being

the turning point in my career. Not only did I sell the work and build long-lasting relationships which generated follow-up work, but that day I found my voice and established myself as a leader. Gone was the self-doubt, the fear, the worry, the self-loathing and other blockages that prevented me from shining brightly. I began trusting myself at this meeting. I spoke eloquently. My mind was clear and words came easily. My heart was open and it felt so good to put myself out there and connect with these talented people in front of me in the room. Sealing a business deal is such a high.

The meeting constituted a turning point in my personal growth as well, because it validated the effectiveness of my diet and self-care routine in making me feel my best, even under stressful circumstances. Instead of pulling an all-nighter to get ready, I chose to focus on my regimen to feel high-energy, confident, attractive, clear-thinking, emotionally connected and attentive to the client, resourceful, innovative and focused. In short, I focused on goal-directed nutrition. Let me teach you.

2.
CHANGE YOUR BRAIN AND YOUR BELIEF SYSTEM

Shifting priorities to focus more intently on yourself and your health may feel downright impossible, or intimidating at best. The busy professionals I've coached throughout my career and those I've interviewed for this book shared concerns about voicing their needs at work for fear of being seen as weak or unfit for duty, which could damage their career advancement. Others felt overwhelmed by their obligations, never-ending to-do lists, and constant rushing to get things done. They couldn't see any wiggle room to begin thinking about a different way of doing things, let alone execute change.

I suspect you may be feeling the same way. I did too, for too long, and eventually had a complete meltdown. I paid the price with my physical, mental and emotional health. But then, as a good Six Sigma practitioner, I dissected my thinking process looking for defects to discover that my own belief system and my brain were at fault. The very root cause of my burnout was not my profession, my employer, my family or anything else. It was my belief system and my brain. I had become stuck in overdrive through an old way of thinking, which no longer served me, and was at the mercy of bad habits.

Change your belief system to let the authentic you take the driver's seat.

Belief systems are essential to explore before embarking on a change management process like goal-directed nutrition, because they are the lexis nexus between our goals and our success reaching them. They either support our quest to reach our goals or make our quest more difficult to undertake. Let me explain. As Karl Woods puts it on his blog: "Your belief system is the actual set of precepts from which you live your daily life, those which govern your thoughts, words, and actions." Beliefs can be limiting your perception of your life, or on the contrary, expanding your horizon.

We all have limiting beliefs that hold us back, generate fear and doubt, make us second-guess our desires and prevent us from pushing the boundaries to create a different reality for ourselves. Here, we are going to examine yours.

Let's start the exploration with a few yes or no questions to get your juices flowing. Then we'll move on to open-ended 'high mileage' questions to explore your beliefs.

Circle whether you agree or disagree with these statements:

I currently feel that my boss or my team would have a lower perception of my abilities if…

…I left work early one night?	(YES)	NO
…I took a longer lunch break?	(YES)	NO
…I came to work a little later so that I can exercise in the morning?	(YES)	NO
…I took a midday nap when I felt tired?	(YES)	NO

Next, explore and list all the beliefs under which you operate without judging yourself; that is the set of precepts from which you live your daily life, those which govern your thoughts, words and actions. I will share my old and new beliefs with you at the end of this chapter.

What are my beliefs in the areas of health and career growth? *(For example, "I believe the only way to success is through working hard" or "I have to work twice as hard as everyone else to get recognized" or "I am overweight because I don't exercise enough.")*

I believe hard work is essential to my success (not everyone's). I believe a career requires dedication/sacrifice + let health slide, work always. Work is crucial & success at work is critical. Health is secondary + possibly manage my emotions through work.

Your belief system can either back you up, point you in the right direction and get you the results you want, or it can be the very reason why you are feeling stuck and miserable.

Looking back at your answers to the yes or no questions above and your list of beliefs, ask yourself:

Where do my beliefs come from?

My father was a sole proprietor and hard worker. My mother and her mother were hard workers. His education as an architect encouraged 'all nighters' and 24 hr work days & 7 day work weeks.

SOMETHING IS OFF ... CLASS seems embedded in My answers

Do I know them to be true? YES / NO

As you embark on the Feeding Success Blueprint, stay open and question what you think you know to be true; question your beliefs. This will be a determining element in your success with GDN and how fast you meet your goals.

What would happen if these beliefs were proven wrong? What would I have the freedom to do that I don't feel I can allow myself today?

I would have a full life — have a life outside work, be connected to others / have a sense of belonging / feel rooted, + have more time; be more relaxed + be more productive + more creative.

It's time to write an alternative set of beliefs for yourself. Beliefs that will support and promote the changes you want to make in your life to break through your personal glass ceiling, to feel great, to look good, and to live the amazing life that has been waiting for you all along.

The new beliefs I would like to live by are...

I work 5-6 hours a day productively
I devote 3-4 hours a day to research / study
I take holidays — true holidays not staycations.
I would like to spend every birthday for the rest of my life in a foreign city
I would like to have few all nighters and not work weekends.
I would like to follow through on my ideas.
I would like to save $, be frugal (but not cheap) and live well!
To live the moment fully
To let the mind go + be ruled by the body more,

Creating a new sets of rules to live by is incredibly hard, but it forces you to think outside the box in terms of what you need to thrive.

It's the difference between whether you enjoy building your career and succeed at it or stress yourself out and become sick over it.

I have worked and resided in four countries: France, my home country; Sweden, where I studied for my MBA and started my professional life; Switzerland and the US. I have also done business in the African, South American and Asian regions. Working in different cultural environments has taught me three things that have been instrumental in changing my belief system and getting me out of 'the matrix'. This mindset shift led me to transform my health and grow my corporate career beyond my wildest dreams.

One. The corporate culture you know is not universal truth. It is bound by the country, company and specific individual or group of people you work with or for. Even if the culture is embedded in laws and policies, as well as unwritten rules, their application can change quite rapidly and how you personally experience them is unique to you.

Two. Thriving in your career and experiencing vibrant health depends on your ability to transcend the status quo, your environment, to find your authentic self and behave in the workplace, at home, and everywhere else, from a place of authenticity and making things work for *you*. When you are authentic, you dare to ask for what you want, to show the real you, without apology. You understand who you are and what you need to thrive, so that you can go get it, which ends up being a win-win for everyone.

what is Corp culture of studio SOMO?

Three. It takes a lot of courage to be authentic. Having the courage to show up and be your authentic self in the eyes of your employer, employees, co-workers, clients and even friends and family stems from a place of self-confidence and self-love, which is more easily achieved when your body, mind and heart are 100% healthy. People who suffer physically, emotionally and mentally tend to hide and protect themselves. They are not authentic because they do not expose their true self, the injured or vulnerable self, to others. What do you think happens then? When you retract and hide, you miss out on the opportunity to genuinely contribute, to be of service to others and make a great impact in the world. You miss out on joy and happiness. Every time you show up being your authentic self, acting, speaking, and thinking with authenticity, you are elevating yourself. You make great strides in the direction of your dreams. You add value. The key to breaking your glass ceiling is to be your fittest and most authentic self.

I am so incredibly excited for you because I know you will succeed. I know how it feels to stand there knowing you're capable of being and doing more, but not knowing how. That is all about to change.

Change your brain to rid yourself of bad habits.

Did you know that 40% of what we do is done out of habit? This is what Charles Duhigg claims in his best-selling book *The Power of Habit: Why We Do What We Do in Life and Business.* When you go get your latte on the way to work in the morning, when you go out to pick up lunch at your favorite deli, when you eat a snack at 3.00pm, when you drink that glass of wine or eat a piece of dark chocolate after dinner, that is habit.

Our habits are deeply rooted in our consciousness. Habits, as neurologists discovered, are patterns inside the brain. In order to successfully change a habit, we need to change our brain. I hear you say: "Easier said than done!" Why is it so hard to change a habit? Because a habit serves a purpose. It is a solution to a problem or a situation that is so effective that it has been hard-wired into our brains. This is powerful stuff, right?

Here's an example. Have you ever tried to stop grabbing lunch out to save some money and lose weight? Maybe you brought your home-cooked lunch into work, but ended up leaving it in the fridge in the office and going out with your co-workers for lunch? Why do you think this habit is so tough to break? What problem does the 'lunching out solution' help you solve?

In my personal experience, lunching out was the only time of the day when I allowed myself to leave the office (go down the 27 floors of the New York skyscraper) and take a breath of fresh air. Bringing my lunch in meant eating at my desk or alone in the pantry with a book or my tablet when everyone else was out having fun.

In order to change that habit of eating out every day, save some money and lose weight, I decided to lunch out with my own food in the spring and summer months at a nearby park with my co-workers. In the fall and winter, my midday time out of the office was replaced by a group fitness class at lunchtime followed by a brief lunch in the pantry.

When traveling, a habit I tried to break was excessive nightly drinking at the hotel bar or during team dinners. I discovered that alcohol was serving two purposes: entertainment when a social dinner was draining my energy; comfort and relaxation when I felt lonely at a hotel bar or after a stressful day. Conquering this bad habit meant reshaping my entire travel lifestyle and dietary habits, which we'll dive into in Part II.

Let's look at your habits. Most of us know what we do wrong, but we don't always fully comprehend why.

Here is a list of all the bad habits that are harming my health and that I wish I could replace or stop indulging in:

- EXERCISE: IRREGULAR PRACTICE; STOP WHEN MOST NEEDED; INCONSISTENT
- RESTING: I DON'T REST WELL; DON'T BREATHE HOLD STRESS
- LUNCH = OFTEN EAT QUICKLY @ COMPUTER on DESK WHEN I COULD GO HOME
- FOOD CHOICES = ARE OFTEN DESTRUCTIVE WHEN EATING OUT & OVER EAT SWEET TOOTH; OFTEN CHOOSE SUGARED OVER NATURAL KNOW WHAT A GOOD DIET CONSISTS OF BUT OFTEN STRAY TOWARD NON-NUTRITIOUS BUT EMOTIONALLY SATISFYING FOOD.
- EARLY RISER BUT INSTEAD OF MEDITATING I MESS OUT EMAILS & CHECK HOROSCOPE AND TEND TO GET WOUND UP & WASTE TIME
- FOCUSING: TENDENCY TO MULTITASK CAN LEAVE ME SCATTERED & PROLONG REACHING GOALS - OR DELAY ENTIRELY
- PROCRASTINATOR! FEAR & LACK OF CLARITY ALLOW ME TO DELAY WORK / ISSUES. AVOID DIFFICULT SUBJECTS / TASKS OFTEN SURPRISED AT EASE ONCE DONE.
- WORRY / FRET RATHER THAN ACT.
- SOCIALIZING = TENDENCY TO SHY AWAY; TO BE WITHDRAWN TRY 22 TO DO TOO MANY THINGS
- LATENESS = DISCOMFORT SITTING IDLE / SOCIALIZIN
- SELF ABSORPTION =

What purpose are these bad habits serving? How do they nurture me emotionally, mentally and possibly physically?

INSECURITIES & FEAR & LACK OF CONFIDENCE

What could I replace these bad habits with to fulfill my needs and nurture my health?

- REGULAR EXERCISE = YOGA DAILY MEDITATION & CARDIO 3x WK.
- REST = BETTER QUALITY, ↑ SLEEP / 8HRS MIN
- ↓ STRESS ALLOW FOR DAY DREAMING / DOWN TIME / CREATIVE PLAY SCHEDULE REGULAR VACATIONS
- RISE EARLY TO GROUND SELF & SET INTENTION BEFORE WORKING. EMAILS AFTER
- TO FOCUS SET GOALS & TASKS AND LIMIT THEM / PRIORITIZE THEM DO NOT JUMP AT EACH PROMPT PRIORITIZE FIRST.
- ARRIVE EARLY AS THIS IS A WAY OF ADDING SPACE & RELAXING
- ACT / DO IT OR DELEGATE IT
- HEALTHY FOOD CHOICES NOW! COOK @ HOME, EAT LUNCH @ HOME OR PACK LUNCH. BE MORE DISCERNING, ↑ NUTRITIONAL VALUE WHEN EATING OUT. IT'S OK TO NOT BE FULL

23

GDN provides you with knowledge and tools to help you design new habits, but being clear on what you do and why you do it is an important first step. Congratulations on completing your self-assessment.

As a former management consultant, I love assessments! They bring clarity on the As-Is situation and inform how much effort is needed to execute an organizational change, to reach the To-Be state. They also inform you of what areas within the business are broken and need revamping. In the next chapter, we'll get clear on where *you* are starting this GDN journey and the challenges you're currently facing.

EMMA'S STORY

I busted several of my beliefs to get unstuck and created new ones to live by. I now understand that, as long as I live, my belief system will need to evolve to support my growth.

Old beliefs included:

- I need to sacrifice my life to have a great career. It's best to work twice as hard in my 20s and 30s as things will slow down as I get older and have a family.

- I need to work beyond the call of duty to show dedication to my career and even harder again in promotion years. As such, I don't have time for a lunch break and me-time. (A calendar filled with lunch meetings or lunch-and-learns would be the closest to a lunch 'off').

- I cannot leave work early (even if I'm done with my work for the day) and I should work two or three weekends a month.

- If I say no to overtime, it will hurt my chances for future advancement and I will never get work again from this partner/director/boss.

- This is still very much a man's world. It is harder to make it to the top of the hierarchy as a woman. I need to work twice as hard as a man to make it.

- I need to have a higher rating than my co-worker in order to get promoted. Basically, I need to beat others to advance, make more money, and have more visibility.

- There are limited positions at such-and-such a level in the company or in certain areas of expertise.

- Carbs will make me fat. I shed more weight with diets higher in lean protein and I need to eat (animal) protein at every meal.

- If I don't exercise as much or more than I eat, I will gain weight.

- I am doing well with six hours sleep during the week and can catch up on sleep over the weekend (so I can keep working late nights, or going out for dinner at 8.00pm with co-workers, clients or my iPad every night on the road).

- Work-life balance is met if I work hard and play hard.

- Companies don't really support work-life balance. That is good marketing but somewhat suspicious. If you are really serious about your career and making it to the top, it does not apply to you.

This belief system went kaput when I burned out and had to go on a two-month medical leave of absence. Hardly the right way to advance a career and promote happiness!

The new belief system I created during my medical leave of absence was a game changer for me. It enabled me to regain my health and move up the career ladder faster to the next level, while lowering stress levels, freeing time for me to go back to school to deepen my understanding of integrative health, and create a start-up.

This is what my new beliefs looked like:

- Killing myself at work is not a prerequisite for success. Hard work can move me up the ladder and earn me more money, but so can ease-filled inspired action.

- As a creative woman, what inspires and motivates me is the desire to achieve things and realize my vision, not competing with others. Through inspiration instead, I can achieve results by knowing I've eliminated the stress of conformity and competition. I am in my own category and the strides I make realizing my vision are what earns me more success, more money, more recognition and an infinite amount of joy. Another derived result of this belief is that it ensures that the work I do, the projects I pick, the companies I chose to give my talent to and the clients I work with are the right fit for me. Those with whom I share my vision will be interested in what I bring to the table. The amount of energy saved by not having to conform and compete is huge!

- Although culturally, the gender dynamics are different in the US to what I experienced working in Sweden, self-achievement is not gender-specific. In fact, we all run both masculine (yang) and feminine (yin) energy within us and constantly choose which energy to emphasize in any given situation. I use a blend of feminine and masculine energy every day by being caring and inclusive (yin), as well as warm, creative, decisive, fearless and action-oriented (yang). Further, success established on my own terms earns me respect and support from male partners, on equal terms. Animosity, rivalry or resentment are not feelings on which to build a positive career foundation.

- Carbs and cheese don't make me fat. Stress, exhaustion, unhappiness and toxic foods do. I lose weight when I sleep eight to nine hours a night, relax more and stress less, exercise less aggressively (not beating myself up), enjoy life, cook homemade meals and eat the highest quality whole foods filled with life force, micro-nutrients and superfoods instead of packaged junk. By comparison, the amount of carbs, protein and fat that I eat are of marginal consideration.

- Freedom is my deepest core desire. I am free to do anything I want in this life and, however far down a path I may have gone, it is never too late to change my mind, turn around and get out of the situation. There is no shame in failure or abandoning a decision, if I navigate my life by the feeling of freedom and being authentic.

- "The point of life is happiness". So said The Dalai Lama. Happiness is my new compass. All the choices I make today are driven by increasing joy and decreasing pain, not by money, power, obligation or someone else's agenda. I believe that pain is a gift from our body, heart and mind asking for change. Suffering however is optional, if we make the required changes! If I feel boredom, sadness, anger, resentment, jealousy, or pain in my body, I listen intently to my emotions and physical self and try to understand what decision I made, activity I did, or words I said to bring about this pain in me.

3.
SELF-ASSESS THE STATE OF YOUR HEALTH

Now that you have set your intentions for change and evaluated your belief system, let's take an honest look at the starting point of your journey.

Excess weight, exhaustion, high blood pressure, high cholesterol, depression, chronic colds, aches and pains, and anything else that is causing you discomfort today is a symptom of an imbalance in your lifestyle and diet.

Our bodies are the perfect computers. They perform thousands of functions per second and don't make mistakes. They try continuously to maintain homeostasis and balance. They digest the wrong foods we feed them and try to make something out of those substances. When we get hurt, our bodies start to heal instantly. They put us to sleep and wake us up every day. In short, our bodies love us. Your body loves you!

However unpleasant it is to acknowledge, we are responsible for a lot of the things that happen to us. Sadly, we're not good at detecting the 'pink flags', those subtle early warnings from our body that something's off, indicating greater health problems in the making ('red flags').

Your body loves you. It loves you so much that it tells you what is wrong very early on. All you need to do is listen and learn your own body's language and cues for balance or lack thereof.

The Goal-Directed Nutrition Circle of Health on the next page is a self-assessment framework to help you intuitively identify the pink flags.

The Goal-Directed Nutrition Circle of Health has 20 sections. Look at each section and place a dot on the segment marking how healthy you are. A dot placed at the center of the circle or close to the middle of the segment indicates dissatisfaction, while a dot placed further out toward the edge of the circle indicates rocking health. When you have placed a dot on each section, connect them to see your Goal-Directed Nutrition Circle of Health. You will have a clear visual of imbalances and a baseline to measure your progress as you embark on The Feeding Success Blueprint.

THE GOAL-DIRECTED NUTRITION CIRCLE OF HEALTH

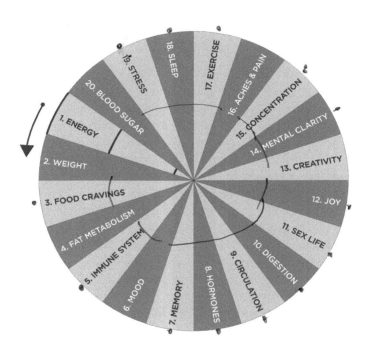

How did your Goal-Directed Nutrition Circle of Health self-assessment come out?

When I first completed the Goal-Directed Nutrition Circle of Health, I was shocked to see how many areas were functioning sub-optimally in my body. Everything but exercise, circulation and my sex life was off. Out of 20 areas, 17 needed remediation! I started to understand the cumulative effect and inter-relatedness of these imbalances.

For instance, I realized how the lack of sleep increased my sugar cravings, which made my blood sugar swing and my mood fluctuate. Lack of sleep also weakened my immune system which led to an increase in the number of colds I would get each year. I also saw the connection between stress, poor digestion, mental fog, lack of creativity and poor concentration. I realized that my back pain and headaches were my liver, kidney and adrenal glands' cry for help. My aches and pains made it hurt to exercise (even though I did until my diagnosis), which further increased my stress, insomnia, and digestive issues. The lack of energy and sleep deprivation made it less fun to be around people, socialize at work or with friends. I was becoming short-tempered with my family, and defensive when receiving constructive feedback at work. I was unhappy, less creative and my forward-thinking suffered. I stopped painting, which was a creative outlet I loved. In the end, this accumulation of seemingly isolated health imbalances over the years led to a massive and systemic breakdown.

The big question then is: what causes such a downfall and how do we reclaim our health or prevent the erosion of it from happening in the first place?

A study published in the *Journal of Occupational and Environmental Medicine* in 2011 showed that people who travel for business two weeks or more a month have poorer health over a number of measurements. They have higher body mass index (BMI), higher rates of obesity, lower HDL cholesterol, higher blood pressure and poorer self-rated health than those who travel less often.

It is difficult to maintain a healthy lifestyle when working long hours pursuing deadlines in the office or being on the road all the time:

- Clean food, fresh fruit and vegetables are generally not available on airplanes and trains, or at airports, train stations and restaurants, although this is changing.

- The office worker and, more so, the business traveler, is chronically dehydrated. Clean water is also not readily available, unless you carry bottled water on you. Tap water isn't always good. Airplane water is of poor quality and more than 20 airlines failed testing against the Environmental Protection Administration (EPA) standards (more on that later). It is also inconvenient to urinate when traveling so we drink less, except of course, the favored 'choices of the business consultant': beer and soda. In the office, meetings are scheduled back to back preventing bathroom breaks, and making us refrain from drinking enough water.

- We tend to over-eat when having breakfast, lunch and dinner out. The food is richer and portions are much bigger. (Who goes for oatmeal when you have a breakfast buffet available?) Takeout is also common late in the evening when the team is working on finishing a project.

- Hard-to-resist snacks, usually the packaged processed kind, are everywhere in the workplace. They are in baskets on conference tables, front desks, vending machines and people's drawers.

- There is peer pressure. Other people will try to coax you back into the unhealthy dining options you are trying to avoid. Change can make others uncomfortable and standing your ground feels like a daring act.

- Even catered lunches and cafeteria food is of poor quality. They rarely include the most important healthy foods. Most offices are located in business parks surrounded by fast-food chains offering no option for a health-promoting meal.

- Busy professionals and business travelers do not cook often enough or at all. According to American survey results published in the *Huffington Post* in 2011, 28% do not know how to cook. Ignorance was the second most cited reason for not cooking regularly and the most cited reason, with 51%, was reliance on the spouse's cooking.

- The amount of wine and liquor consumed on business trips between happy hour, dining out with co-workers and clients, and waiting at the airport lounge or on the plane exceeds the acceptable one glass per day.

- It is harder to sleep when eating dinner late, drinking alcohol, sleeping in a strange hotel bed, hearing unfamiliar noises, and dealing with jetlag. God forbid you are taking an overnight flight weekly...

- It is more difficult to get into an exercise routine when traveling, when the day is never-ending and you feel chronically fatigued.

- There is little room to unwind on the road as the stress relievers available back home, like family support, visiting a friend, going to see a play or working out, may not be available.

- On the road, trying to have me-time almost feels like slacking. It is not a vacation trip but a business trip, with a perception that time on site, collocated with the client or team needs to be maximized.

With high stress levels and low energy, processed food and liquor become the recreational drugs that numb the pain of the overworked business professional and power us through the day or night. Both are addictive. And dangerous. In fact, 90% of current health issues such as obesity, diabetes, heart disease and cancer have been linked to the poor quality of the processed food we eat and a poor lifestyle.

Now assess yourself.

What are the top three behaviors that derail my health when I travel and get caught up in my busy workday?

_____
_____
_____
_____
_____
_____
_____
_____

How does having poor health make me feel? *(Sluggish, tired, foggy mind, depressed, heavy, unmotivated, unhappy, poor self-confidence, etc.)*

_____

_____

_____

_____

_____

_____

_____

_____

How does my poor health affect others around me in my life?

_____

_____

_____

_____

_____

_____

_____

_____

What are three things that I could start doing to improve my health and happiness today?

_____

_____

_____

_____

_____

_____

In the next chapter, we'll begin to look at the solution with an introduction to the power of food and the principles behind goal-directed nutrition.

4.
THE FIVE PRINCIPLES OF GOAL-DIRECTED NUTRITION

Goal-directed nutrition (GDN) is an approach I've developed over the last 10 years of my project and change management consulting career as my nutrition and fitness practice was maturing. My education and professional experience in both fields have grown on parallel tracks since my very first year of college in France.

Goal-directed nutrition was inspired by a project management methodology that I'm very fond of and have practiced for years called goal-directed project management. It was originally developed by Coopers and Lybrand in Europe in the 1980s. The methodology is very results-focused and allows for flexibility and continuous refinement in project execution, with the project details getting more and more refined as the goals are closer to being met. Goal-directed project management is centered around the breakdown of goals and objectives, setting project milestones, and organizing, developing and aligning people with the systems being implemented in the organization.

I like to think of goal-directed nutrition as the intersection of people, food and lifestyle, including support systems, which enables you to get the results you want, to reach your goals. The big idea behind GDN is that when you fuel your body and your mind in the right way, you become the best version of yourself. This can help you reach your other goals in life and business faster and with more enjoyment. Being healthy creates a ripple effect of success in all other areas of your life, including your career. The reverse is also true: a deteriorating heath eventually cripples your career, the pleasure you receive from your work and your relationships.

Now, this idea may sound a little 'out there' for most of us driven business professionals. I didn't think about food as a powerful agent of change myself until I became sick and started to learn about Traditional Chinese Medicine and Ayurveda, which are thousands of years old, but still very much in use in the US and the rest of the world today. I became passionate about the topic when I experienced first-hand how changing my diet and lifestyle also changed the way I felt and performed.

Being born and raised in France, my relationship with food was always one driven by pleasure and childhood memories of long family lunches or dinners with four lavish courses (not including the *aperitif* drinks with *petits-fours* and *digestif* drinks and sweets). From my grandmother's *canard à l'orange* (orange-glazed duck) to my aunt's *petits choux* (profiteroles), my uncle's famous cheese platter, Papa's freshly caught wild oysters and my mum's *foie gras,* I have been well-raised on the *art de la table.* I grew up in Bordeaux, my university facing the vineyards of Pessac-Leognan. Wine and gourmet food were and still are passions of mine. My sweet spot is how to make gourmet healthier.

But what I discovered was that, to survive their pace of life, busy professionals and business travelers need to eat differently than they would when relaxing on Sunday or on vacation. Even us French!

The diet of the busy professional is one that supports his health under pressure. Excess wine, heavy meals, too much animal saturated fat, too few fresh vegetables and fruit, too much stress, too little exercise, and routine sleep deprivation means sickness is a not-so-distant reality.

Traditional Chinese Medicine and Ayurveda have long used the power of food (animal, vegetables, fruit, herbs, roots) and food energetics to cure people's illnesses, strengthen the body and balance the mind. Modern pharmaceuticals mimic nature's wonders too, by extracting compounds from food to make pills. So why wouldn't food, which already contains so many known (and unknown) compounds, not work just as well if not more effectively than a pill? As it has in 5,000 years of ancient wisdom and medical tradition. Having researched, learned and experimented on myself, brought my conditions under control, energized my life and boosted my career, you might say I'm a convert!

Goal-directed nutrition is a blueprint based on my experience, as well as my learnings from the work of prominent doctors, scientists, nutritionists, botanists and spiritual leaders. Indeed, during my training at the Institute for Integrative Nutrition®, I studied over 100 dietary theories, practical lifestyle management techniques, and innovative coaching methods with some of the world's top health and wellness experts. My teachers included Dr. Andrew Weil, Director of the Arizona Center for Integrative Medicine; Dr. Deepak Chopra, leader in the field of mind-body medicine; Dr. David Katz, Director of Yale University's Prevention Research Center; Dr. Walter Willett, Chair of Nutrition at Harvard University; Dr. T Colin Campbell, the Jacob Gould Schurman Professor Emeritus of Nutritional Biochemistry at Cornell University and author of *The China Study*; Geneen Roth, bestselling-author and expert on emotional eating; and many other leading researchers and nutrition authorities.

I am not a doctor. I am a board-certified health and nutrition coach, with many fitness certifications and experience in the business world as a director of a management consulting firm (not to mention first-hand experience of the toll taken by thousands of frequent flyer miles).

My intention with GDN is to distill and present to you how food and lifestyle can help you become the shining star in your life and the lives of others around you, and prevent chronic fatigue, burnout and sickness.

EMMA'S STORY

Like you, I have been a driven and busy professional all my adult life. I have been dedicated to my consulting work, volunteered time to community service and charity events, held leadership positions in global professional associations (such as the Project Management

Institute), and spent another 20 hours a week in my fitness and nutrition hobby. I know first-hand what it feels like to juggle tasks all day and live out of a suitcase.

I also know what it feels like to be chronically fatigued and sick. As I was making dietary and lifestyle changes, not only did my health improve but both my careers, in consulting and in wellness, exploded. I attracted the best clients, exponentially increased my network and, on a personal front, I met the love of my life and bought my dream house.

I believe that success at work and in life starts with the food you eat. For this reason, I would like to frame nutrition in your mind and clear up some confusion caused by all the contradictory information out there.

Like any good theory, GDN comes with a set of principles to guide your understanding and exploration of that theory. GDN's five principles will extend your knowledge of the types of food available for you to eat, the effects of these foods on your physical and psychological being, why you should eat them, as well as fostering a deeper knowledge of your own body and personal limitations.

The foods recommended in GDN are not designed with a political or spiritual agenda, as is the case with other dietary theories that ban certain foods, like meat for instance. If there were to be an agenda, I'd say mine was to provide you with a guide to reclaim your health, increase your energy, create and strengthen your emotional stability and mental acumen amidst a busy professional life and stressful business travel schedule, because I've been there and I know what it's like.

And your health does not have to suffer the way mine did.

Here are the five GDN guiding principles:

PRINCIPLE I
FOOD IS INFORMATION FOR YOUR BODY: EAT HIGH QUALITY NUTRIENT-DENSE WHOLE FOODS.

Food is more than the sum of its calories and grams of carbohydrates, protein and fat. Food is information for your body. It tells your body how to express its genes, which genes to turn on and off. Natural foods, especially wholesome and organic choices, are alive. They contain enzymes and a variety of organic and inorganic compounds (vitamins, minerals, phytonutrients), which enable the body to function most optimally. Did you know that 95% of your body's functions depend on minerals? To paraphrase David Wolfe, the raw food guru, your health and beauty depends on the mineralization of your body. So my first advice to you is to make sure these foods are the star of your meals.

Here's what you need to know. Simply stated, food is made of macro-nutrients (carbohydrates, fat and protein), micro-nutrients (organic compounds like vitamins, and inorganic compounds like minerals and phytonutrients), dietary fiber, cholesterol (only in animal food) and enzymes.

Every nutrient in the food you eat is coded with a purpose. It provides information to your tissues and your organs. It triggers a reaction at the cellular level.

The vitamins and minerals contained in the food you eat are essential for life and responsible for your body's metabolic functions. The body deciphers the coded purpose of each substance and uses it accordingly. For instance, iron is the foundation of the hemoglobin molecule, which carries oxygen from the lungs to the cells in the body. Vitamin D promotes the absorption and use of calcium and phosphate for healthy bones and teeth. Potassium is essential to maintain proper fluid balance, nerve impulse function, muscle function and cardiac (heart muscle) function. In fact, every micro-nutrient serves a role in your body. Chronic deficiency in micro-nutrients will break down your body and threaten your life.

Eating whole foods containing the highest *micro-nutrient density* (to use a term coined by Dr. Joel Fuhrman in his book *Eat To Live*) provides the most robust foundation for your health.

The most important factor for optimal health, increased energy and weight loss is that you consume a diet with a high *nutrient-per-calorie ratio*. As such, gauge a food by the amount of micro-nutrients it provides you, rather than counting calories for the sake of counting calories or obsessing on getting 'enough' grams of protein, carbs and fats. Start counting micro-nutrients and eat the protein, carbs and fats that provide you with highest amount of those micro-nutrients. Through the lens of micro-nutrition density, all protein, carbs and fat are not created equal and cannot be compared in terms of calories and grams.

Let's look at protein first. Protein is used for the manufacturing of every cell in your body, the regulation of enzymes and hormones, for growth, for the structure of your blood cells and for the functioning of antibodies. The source and quantity of the protein you ingest determines the quality of your build, tissue growth and resistance to infection.

From the lens of nutrient-density, a 100 calories serving of beef and a 100 calories serving of broccoli looks very different, as shown in tables comparing nutrient-density of various foods in Dr. Fuhrman's *Eat To Live* book and website.

Indeed, 100 calories of broccoli contains more calcium, iron, magnesium, potassium, vitamins A, C, E, folate, niacin, riboflavin and even protein than beef (11g against 6g for sirloin steak) and a near equal amount of zinc. The serving of broccoli also contains fiber, high levels of phytochemicals, antioxidants and beta-carotene which are completely missing in the serving of beef. Lastly, broccoli contains none of the saturated fat and cholesterol present in meat. The only things going for meat, except the taste and vitamin B12 (not often present in plant fare), is that beef is protein-dense: 100 calories of beef is less voluminous (1oz) than 100 calories of broccoli (12.6oz). However, if your primary intake of protein is animal food like beef, pork and chicken, you are lacking crucial micro-nutrients to promote your health. The solution? Vary your intake of protein to increase the spectrum and amount of micro-nutrients consumed.

The same concept of nutrient density and quality is true of fats and carbohydrates. All fats and carbohydrates are not created equal. Catchy magazine titles saying "low fat diets may prevent cancer and heart disease" or "low carb diets may accelerate weight loss" fail to mention the importance of quality and how the right kinds of fats and carbohydrates will actually help you lose weight faster, and prevent disease. Cutting the good fats and carbohydrates out of your diet would in fact be detrimental to your health and weight loss efforts as they contain essential micro-nutrients. A sign that popular beliefs and those of the medical community are starting to change and that fat may not be something to fear or ban at all costs is the article "Ending the War on Fat" in *Time Magazine* dated June 12, 2014, which finally acknowledges that saturated fat does not cause heart disease and that real butter is better than margarine.

Indeed, fats are necessary to protect your body's tissues and organs, maintain your body's temperature, enable conversion of fat-soluble vitamins (A, D, E and K). Fats are also a good source of fuel and prevent dryness and dehydration in the body. Helpful to conserve a youthful appearance when you work in an air-conditioned office and travel weekly in pressurized airplanes, don't you think? The type and quality of the fat you ingest, whether saturated, polyunsaturated or mono-unsaturated, will determine how well these functions will be met. The micro-nutrient density profile of lard, butter, olive oil, coconut oil, nuts and avocado vary greatly.

Carbohydrates provide an excellent source of long-lasting energy. However, their systemic effect on your body will differ based on which types you're consuming. Simple sugars (monosaccharides and disaccharides from fruit, milk, or candy) and complex carbohydrates (polysaccharides and oligosaccharides found in wholegrain cereal, root vegetables and legumes) will provide different information to your body.

There is one more factor to consider when choosing the most nutrient-dense foods. Nutrient density is also affected by the way the food you eat was grown, distributed and prepared. And you cannot fully trust the nutrition labels to determine that. Here's why. The nutritional information on wholewheat pasta enriched with vitamins and minerals could appear the same on the package as that of a wholewheat grain, but the quality of their nutrition and effect on the body would be drastically different.

Compare wholewheat pasta, made from pulverized whole wheat, with the wholewheat grain, which contains the bran, germ and endosperm. As shown in the Wikipedia drawing replica, the more nutrient-dense part of the wheat, including the fiber, is found in the bran and the germ which are destroyed during the pulverization of the grain to make it into the flour required for manufacturing pasta. The germ is removed because polyunsaturated fats can make the flour rancid, shortening the product's shelf-life. As a result, synthetic vitamins and minerals have to be added back in by the manufacturer to increase the nutritional value of the food. From the research I've read, it is unclear whether the body recognizes or is able to utilize synthetic vitamins and minerals efficiently. So which would you prefer to eat?

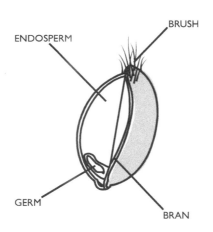

	Carb /g	Protein /g	Fat /g	Fiber /g	Iron (% daily req.)	Others
Bran	63	16	3	43	59	vitamin Bs
Endosperm	79	7	0	4	7	
Germ	52	23	10	14	35	vitamin Bs omega-3/6 lipids

These two products cannot be considered to be the same quality, even though the amount of macro- and micro-nutrients appear the same on the nutritional label. Further, their effect on the body will be totally different; flour products such as bread and pasta create an immediate spike in blood sugar and insulin release, while whole grains deliver a more moderate and continuous release of blood sugar, providing sustainable energy over a longer period of time.

Knowing where your food comes from and how it was prepared will enable you to choose more wisely and eat the most nutrient-dense and health-promoting foods while limiting the less healthy options.

Taking into account the information makeup of the food you eat and choosing the most nutrient-dense foods is the first foundational principle of GDN.

PRINCIPLE 2
FOOD IS ENERGY AND AFFECTS HOW YOU FEEL: EAT THE FOODS THAT MAKE YOU FEEL YOUR VERY BEST.

The second principle may come as a surprise to you if you've considered food as merely a way to fuel your physical body. Food is fuel and information, but there is more to food than its nutritional attributes.

Food also affects *how you feel.* The magic of food resides in its energetic power. This may seem far-fetched to you, but the concept of 'food energetics', as it's called, has been around for thousands of years in ancient wisdom traditions. More recently, Steve Gagné, a natural health and nutrition counselor, studied and described it in his excellent book *Food Energetics: The Spiritual, Emotional, and Nutritional Power of What We Eat.*

In it, Steve explains that each food has an essential character and temperament, and that when we eat that food, its energy travels through very specific, pre-determined pathways throughout our bodies and correlate with our human mind and body.

Thinking about that, all things being equal in terms of calories, the energy you feel from eating beef, fish, quinoa, kale or apple feels completely different. If you want to live a high-energy life and reduce physical, mental and emotional stress, you need to eat the foods that make you feel that way, and establish a lifestyle that creates and saves energy. If you feel tired all the time, the food you eat, the exercise routine you follow, your sleep schedule, the relationships you may be engaged in, and any other lifestyle attributes may not be right for you.

Too few people connect what they eat to the desired outcomes in their lives. By understanding food energetics, you will be able to use food beyond its nutritional power to control your energy, enhance your health and achieve top performance. Food will be your secret weapon to making it to the top and staying there!

EMMA'S STORY

Food energetics has been a game-changer for me and it enabled me to transform my life. I use food to balance my moods and control my stress levels. I use food to calm me down and induce restful sleep. I use food to ground me and increase my focus, to energize me, to enhance my self-confidence, to make me feel euphoric, to cool me down, to warm me up, to relax me and fire me up. I also learned how to use food energetics to reboot certain internal organs and systems, especially when they were affected by stress. In particular, I'm thinking of my digestive system, including my GI tract, liver and kidneys, my endocrine system and my cardiovascular system. I will show you which foods to use to temper your busy and stressed life.

How does food energetics work? Here is what you need to know in order to experience its magic for yourself:

One. Food quality is paramount. The energetics of food, which emanates from the essential nature of food, can only be experienced with real food of superior quality, as in naturally grown plants and naturally raised animal food. Food processing, genetic alteration or conventionally grown foods (which are altered with chemicals) denature the food of its identity and strip it of its energy. Processed foods do not travel through specific pathways. Their energetics and information power is diminished in processing.

Two. Foods have an essential character. A cow is a cow and not a chicken. Although you can get protein from the cow and the chicken (or from vegetables), the cow has its own unique makeup of amino acids and other nutrients that makes it a cow and nothing else. By extension, no other food has the same nutritional profile as beef. When trying to understand and use food energetics, comparative nutrition profiling is misleading. The very purpose of studying food energetics is to get to know the uniqueness of each food in order to select the right food for the right energetic effect. The essential character of a food is what gives it its unique identity as kale, chicken, carrot, nuts and so on.

There are four essential characters in food energetics as I learned from Steve Gagné in nutrition school:

- 'Up and out': A plant that grows upwards and spreads its leaves outwards, like broad leafy greens (chard, collard greens, lettuce, leafy bok choy), or fruit from vines or trees like grapes and peaches.

- 'Up and in': A plant that grows upwards towards the sky and has a more drying, purging and tightening effect on the body, like the bitter leafy greens kale, dandelion greens, mustard greens, and chives.

- 'Down and out': Plants that grow close to the earth or underneath it and expand on the soil outwards, like a potato, onion and turnip.

- 'Down and in': Plants that grow deep underground, with greater penetrating quality and more intense absorption of soil nutrients and water, like carrots and burdock roots.

What is fascinating about this study on the characteristics of various foods is that foods correlate with the various characteristics of our own body and mind.

As such, foods with upward energy relate to our upper body such as our circulatory and respiratory functions (throat, lungs, heart), while the foods with downward energy relate to the lower body such as the digestive and reproductive systems (intestines, colon, bladder, sexual organs). There are also foods where energy correlates with the organs in the middle of the body (liver, gallbladder, spleen, pancreas, stomach, kidneys).

For example, a carrot has a 'down and in' nature. It grows deep 'down' buried into the earth and absorbs 'in' all the water and nutrients from the soil. In our body, an organ presenting the same 'down and in' character is the small intestine, where most of the food is absorbed through the villi into the blood stream. On the other hand, dark leafy greens, like Swiss chard or kale, with their green leaves and complex veins, remind us of our own lungs and circulatory system. They have an upward energy and help strengthen and purify our blood, clear congestion and mucus in our lungs, building our internal rainforest, our center of life.

Interestingly, Graves' disease (with its first manifestation in the throat, eyes and heart) called for more foods with an upward energy which were mostly unaccounted for on my business traveler's diet. A diet which was also plagued by unnatural chemically processed foods and beverages. (Sigh.)

Three. Foods have a temperament. Keep an open mind here. In food energetics, foods also have psychological attributes called temperament. Just like we human beings can be described as being 'hot-blooded', 'warm', 'cool', 'cold-blooded', foods can be categorized in four temperaments: hot, cold, warm and cool. Each of these temperaments are further qualified as dry or damp. Foods can therefore be classified as hot and damp (beef), warm and dry (chicken), cool and damp (trout), warm and damp (almonds, kidney beans), cold and dry (long grain rice), cold and damp (lettuce leaf), etc.

From a psychological standpoint, eating a carrot (warm and damp) buried in the earth will make us feel grounded and rooted. I've snacked on baby carrots for years to help me overcome my anxiety of public speaking. Chewing slowly on carrots before important client presentations or public speaking engagements has helped me combat nervousness and settle my gut. Carrots, because of their 'down, in and warm' nature, invariably comfort and center me. They have a relaxing and calming effect on my digestive system.

On the other hand, eating the Swiss chard or kale has an uplifting energetic effect. Leafy greens promote a subtle, light and flexible energy in our body and increase creativity and emotional stability.

Now, thinking about the temperament of food described above, which character and temperament do you think you have? Are you hot or cold? Warm or cool? Damp or dry? Give it some thought for a minute.

_____

_____

_____

_____

_____

_____

_____

Many busy professionals I worked with tended to be the 'hot and damp' kind, harboring a strong type A personality. Many were controlling and had a temper, as well as a physical tendency to overheat and sweat profusely. The other proportion were 'hot and dry', projecting dominance without the outburst of passion!

Another temperament I find quite prevalent in New York City is the 'cold and dry' type. This person works very hard (too hard) to stay in shape and fears fat. 'Cold and dry' people tend not to eat enough lubricating fats and are at risk of physical deficiencies, eating disorders, and emotional struggles with fear, insecurity, guilt and depression.

What foods do you think would worsen each of these temperaments, for instance? Yes! The hot and damp foods for the former and the cold and dry foods for the latter.

There are many variations of characters and temperaments. Understanding yours and knowing the states of balance and imbalance is an important step in your journey of using food energetics to feel better.

Four. Food preparation affect the energetics of food. The food temperament is affected by food preparation and cooking methods. As you most likely know, chemical changes occur during food preparation and cooking. Upon heating your food, for instance, its texture changes, its smell changes, some nutrients disappear, while others become more digestible. In food energetics, different food preparation and cooking techniques will affect the energy of the food in different ways and affect the way you feel:

- Cooking techniques that have an upward and rising energy, which help you feel light, creative and flexible include blanching, boiling, quick water sautéing, quick pressing, quick marinating, juicing and raw foods.

- Cooking techniques that have an downward energy and help you feel grounded and relaxed include stewing, pressure cooking and baking.

- Cooking techniques and foods that make you feel tense, nervous, anxious and angry include: microwave cooking, electric stove cooking (unlike gas cooking) and using/eating foods tainted with chemicals and hormones (factory farming, GMO foods, etc.)

Five. The seasons affect the energetics of food and your body's needs. Eating in season is another key factor when considering the energetics of food and what your body requires in order to thrive. Basically, eating foods in season increases the energetic power of your food. Think of tomatoes, for instance. You can find tomatoes all year round because of importation and greenhouses, but tomatoes are at their energetic peak when they are at their ripest, deepest red and most aromatic with lots of flesh, which is in the late summer. Eating food at its energetic peak results in a greater concentration of nutrients and a more portent post-digestion effect of the food on your body. Remember, food energetics correlates with the needs of our human body and mind.

In the ancient traditions of TCM and Ayurveda, food is the remedy of the season, like an antidote for the season to supports your body's most active organs during that season. Eating seasonally will therefore help you feel your best and free your energy, which you can use towards a more productive life.

Here's an example. In the spring, the weather is cold, rainy and damp. The foods harvested in the spring are foods that are diuretic, bitter and astringent and help the body drain the excess fat accumulated over the freezing winter months and rid itself of excess dampness: sprouts, asparagus, artichokes, and bitter and astringent leafy greens like dandelion, mustard greens, spinach, watercress and spring lettuce. The central regulating organ for fat metabolism is the liver. Also prominent is the gallbladder, which creates bile to dissolve fats during digestion. The liver and gallbladder with their rising (upwards) energy are at their most active in the spring and need to be supported by the foods in season for maximum efficiency.

The same is true for the summer, fall and winter months. If you keep eating foods out of season, or the same food all year long—that same old turkey sandwich on wholewheat bread with soup or mesclun salad on the side, that same dinner every night of meat, or chicken, or salmon with a side of broccoli, spinach or potato—you have been missing out on the magic of seasonal eating and how much better your health could be, however fit you are today.

It is especially hard for frequent business travelers eating and dining in airplanes and at the airport where the food menus are standardized and designed to increase shelf-life, portability and ease of consumption, and satisfy the general population's taste buds. Your body's needs change with the season, just like the food that comes to maturity in that season. Learning what to eat and where to find it will be explored in Part II.

Six. Balancing the yin and yang qualities in foods and lifestyle. I'd like to leave you with one last perspective on the energetics of food by taking a look at the ancient Chinese philosophy of yin and yang. This concept may become a very useful tool for you to better manage your energy and understand and control your food cravings. (We all experience them!)

Have you heard of the concept of yin and yang? This ancient understanding defines how the universe is organized into opposite, yet complementary forces. As described by Joshua Rosenthal, founder and director of the Institute for Integrative Nutrition, in his book, *Integrative Nutrition: Feed Your Hunger For Health And Happiness:* "The yang embodies the masculine qualities of hard, strong, active, right and contractive. The yin embodies the feminine qualities of soft, yielding, passive, receptive, loose and expansive."

This concept of opposition and complimentary yin-yang applies to foods as much as it applies to lifestyle, and overlaps the food energetics theory described above. The idea is that to recover and maintain optimum mental, emotional and physical health, you simply need to try to balance your intake of yin foods with yang foods and balance your involvement in yin-type activities with yang-type activities.

Why does it matter? Because too much yin food will make you feel hyper, spacey, nervous, stressed out and, digestion-wise, experience loose stools (useful cue!). Too much yang food will make you feel lethargic, lazy, heavy, depressed, compressed, constricted (constipated) and hardly get anything done. With the right yin-yang balance, you'll feel grounded and uplifted at the same time and your body will function more optimally, with a normal digestion process to confirm it.

Here are examples of foods and lifestyle activities with yin and yang qualities.

MORE YANG

FOOD ⬆ LIFE

FOOD	LIFE
Sea salt	Left Side of the Brain
Eggs	Active, Creative, Hard
Miso and Soy Sauce	Ascend Energy
Red Meat	Aggression
Cheese	Hot and Dry
Poultry	Sunny and Light
	Intense Cardio Workouts
Fish	Weight Lifting
Grains	Stress
Sea Vegetables	

BALANCE POINT

Beans	Right Side of the Brain
Roots & Winter Squash	Passive, Receptive, Soft
Leafy Greens	Depression
Tofu	Descend Energy
Local Fruit	Cold and Wet
Nightshade Vegetables	Shady and Dark
	Restorative yoga, Sun-saluting
Nuts and Seeds	Tai Chi
Tropical Fruit	Qi Kong
Oil	Some dance & Martial Arts
Dairy	Stretching
Honey & Spices ⬇	Meditation

MORE YIN

Finding your healthy balance between a yang lifestyle made of stress, competition, hard deadlines, and a lot of creative left brain work, with yin activities such as meditation, yoga and yin foods is an art. You now have a lot of information to start creating a high-performing diet and lifestyle for yourself using the special energies of food and activities.

PRINCIPLE 3
YOU ARE WHAT YOU EAT, DIGEST AND DON'T EXCRETE: NURTURE YOUR DIGESTIVE AND ELIMINATION SYSTEM FOR RENEWAL.

Every food you eat is either a trigger for better health or a trigger for disease. The food you eat becomes your cells, your organs, your hormones, your blood, your skin, your hair, your bones, and even your thoughts and emotions. Eat clean foods and you'll feel and look better. Eat junk foods and you'll grow old and sick faster, think junk thoughts, and feel emotionally confused.

Would you eat and live differently or treat yourself better, if you were given a new heart, new skin, new bones and new organs?

Your body is younger than you think. You're in luck! You can have new and improved body parts! Did you know that parts of your body are only a few days old, others just a few weeks and months old? In fact, only your eyes (except the cornea) and your brain (excluding the olfactory bulb and hippocampus) are as old as the age shown on your ID.

Given proper nutrition and rest, your body's renewed cells will make you feel reborn. Here are some amazing facts about your body that I hope will give you hope, faith and motivation to change:

- Your heart can renew two to three times over your lifetime.

- Your skeleton is a mix of new and older bones of various densities with the oldest bone being 10 years old.

- Your red blood cells wear out every four months.

- Your liver can renew and regrow itself in five months if surgically ablated.

- Your lungs steadily renew themselves over the course of a year.

- Your hair grows about a one third of an inch each month and the lifespan of one hair is three years for men and six years for women.

- The surface layer of your skin is renewed on average every three weeks.

- Your intestinal lining, the villi, renews in only two to three days. This is really incredible, given that our gut makes up for 70% of our immune system and is continuously under attack from poor quality food, pollution, stomach acid and stress.

- My favorite renewal fact is that of our taste buds. Your taste buds are only 10 days old. This is great news if you have food cravings or are addicted to sugar, salt, bread, cheese, or soda. Three weeks of clean eating following GDN will considerably alter your taste buds and make the old food taste less appealing. It may just kick out the sugar junkie in you!

You now understand why making the right food choices consistently, every day, can lend you a great physique and a disease-free body. So the famous saying goes: "You really are what you eat". I prefer saying: "You are what you eat, digest and don't excrete", because if your digestive and elimination systems are impaired, your transformation will not be as successful.

Eating clean foods may not always feel right, however. There may be some clean natural foods that provide you with digestive issues, in which case, you will not benefit from them. Digestive issues such as bloating, gas, constipation, diarrhea and acid reflux compromise your body's absorption and elimination process. An impaired digestion leads to malnourishment and nutrient deficiency. An impaired elimination process increases your risk of disease, and vulnerability to viruses, bacteria and infections.

A healthy digestion process already consumes a lot of energy, a compromised digestion saps your energy even more. (Have you ever experienced the 3.00pm energy slump?) It also disturbs your sleep, affects your performance during exercise, and of course impacts your concentration at work.

There are many reasons for digestive discomfort and two-thirds of my clients report some kind of digestion or elimination issues. The foods you are eating may not be right for you (allergies or intolerance); the way you prepare your food may be inadequate (under-cooked, overcooked, poor food combination, etc.); you may suffer from a nutrient deficiency (especially magnesium); your digestive organs may be weak, overwhelmed or congested (liver, kidneys, stomach, intestines, colon); you may have secretion imbalances (mucus, hormones and enzymes); you may be affected by side effects from medications; you may have a poor lifestyle or lack exercise; you might lack hydration; you could have a need to fight bacteria overgrowth or infection; and your emotions may be getting in the way of a smooth digestion as well.

Indeed, we know that emotions like sadness, fear, anxiety and stress negatively affect digestion. As you can see, the digestive system is more than the stomach and the intestines. It does not act alone and needs the support of other key organs, as well as the endocrine system and the nervous system. It takes a village, as they say. And a lot can and does go wrong for the busy professional living under stress.

The other key element of a healthy body is a healthy elimination process. Your body knows how to digest natural foods and what to use them for. The right foods for you are digested easily and excreted as waste in the form of urine, sweat and feces. The body's excretion is primarily made of metabolic waste and undigested food residue (fiber). The trouble with processed and contaminated foods is that the body has a hard time ridding itself of their toxicity. So even when you stop eating them, you are not completely out of the woods. The chemicals present in artificial sweeteners, pesticides, preservatives, artificial colorings, so called 'natural' flavoring, chlorine, cadmium and heavy metals like mercury remain, for the most part, trapped in your body's tissues, organs and fat cells for decades, resulting in serious health issues down the road.

The conclusion to all this is simple: the foundation of building a healthy and high-performing you relies as much upon eating the right foods as upon caring for your digestive and elimination health.

As you read on, GDN's dietary guidelines will teach you how to increase your intake of clean food, avoid toxic processed foods, and discuss ways in which you can enhance your digestion and elimination processes, including how to rid your body of toxins that could be taxing your health.

Re-establishing your digestive balance and suddenly increasing your energy will be the first clues that the food you're eating and the lifestyle changes you're making are right for you and that you are progressing.

Think about your own experience. Identify the foods that...

...you digest easily and make you feel light and cheery:

_____

_____

_____

...make you feel sluggish or foggy:

_____

_____

_____

...give you gas and indigestion:

_____

_____

_____

...constipate you:

_____

_____

_____

...give you diarrhea, heartburn or other signs of inflammation:

_____

_____

_____

...increase your hunger levels:

_____

_____

_____

...lower your hunger levels:

_____

_____

_____

...make you feel satisfied and happy:

_____

_____

_____

PRINCIPLE 4
NUTRITION GOES BEYOND THE FOOD: FEED YOURSELF WITH NON-EDIBLE FORMS OF NOURISHMENT FOR OPTIMAL HEALTH.

Your body feeds your mind and your mind feeds your body. Therefore, what nourishes your mind nourishes your body; what nourishes your body nourishes your mind. It's interesting how the relationship goes both ways. The cleaner, stronger, and healthier your body is, the sharper your brain and the more intuitive and emotionally connected you become. And vice versa.

An illustration of the body-mind connection is the relationship between your brain and your gut. Have you ever had 'a gut feeling'? Have you ever felt 'nauseous' in front of certain stressful situation at work? Have you ever had 'butterflies' in your stomach when experiencing elation and anticipation?

The brain can signal the mouth to salivate and the stomach to prepare gastric acid before the food gets there. A distressed stomach can be the result of an anxious, confused or stressed-out mind, or it can cause the mind to feel anxious, confused and stressed.

Intuition is said to reside in your gut. When your digestive system is strong, your sense of intuition is very developed. You can make decisions trusting your gut feelings. When you suffer from digestive issues, you may feel more doubtful, hesitant, distant, skeptical and mistrustful of others. It is much harder to have a hunch or make decisions. Self-confidence and charisma stems from a healthy body. New thoughts and ideas emerge from healthy brain cells.

In order to feed yourself for success, you need to establish a diet and lifestyle that not only fuels your body but also nurtures your mind, and the emotional, spiritual and consciousness part of you.

What really nourishes us, as humans, is a life filled with nurturing relationships (love, friendship, intimacy); an occupation we love and that brings us purpose; a form of exercise we enjoy and that makes us feel good; a consciousness practice (mindfulness, spirituality) to connect with the self and others. What fulfills us can take many forms, but it is what we live for. A healthy body enables us to enjoy our life to the fullest. The healthier we are, the more enjoyment and passion we get from our lives, and the more success we attract.

Think of a time when you were working on a project you were passionate about. So passionate about, in fact, that you lost your appetite or forgot to sleep because of it. You were feeding off your passion for that project. This is what nutrition beyond food is all about.

Another great example has to do with relationships. Think of a time when you fell in love with someone and how you lost your appetite in the midst of the excitement for days and weeks on end.

Equally essential is the need to identify where we are deprived of such nourishment, because lacking exercise, fulfilling relationships, a spiritual practice or a job we love can negatively affect our well-being.

Can you think of a toxic relationship in your life and how miserable it makes you feel? Can you identify the emotional, mental and physical ramifications of such stress on yourself?

Over the following chapters, GDN will introduce you to methods to condition your brain beyond the food so that it supports your body and your digestive process, instead of causing it harm. It will also challenge you to reassess your relationships and make changes in your personal and professional network to build a support system.

These recommendations will likely be the most challenging aspects of the GDN approach to put into practice, but they are the most essential. While the food will condition your body and mind to a great extent, and help you develop self-confidence and inner strength, the changes you make in your lifestyle and relationships will seal the deal.

PRINCIPLE 5
YOUR BLUEPRINT TO HEALTH AND SUCCESS IS BIO-
INDIVIDUAL.

The last GDN principle is that of bio-individuality. This means that there is no one pathway to health and no one way to eat that fits everyone. What your body and mind needs is very much your own unique blueprint. There is no 'average' or 'typical' man or woman. We all differ biochemically, hormonally, genetically, physically, and even in our aspirations for our life, career and happiness. Experts in nutrition are starting to recognize that there is merit in individualizing people's diets and that generic governmental standards, such as the United States Department of Agriculture's MyPlate, may not work for everyone, having been developed for an hypothetical 'average' person.

Bio-individuality also provides a basis for us to understand why so many dietary theories appear contradictory. Veganism, macrobiotics, the Zone Diet, the South Beach Diet, the Paleo Diet, the Atkins Diet, and so on have their merits. They work for some, but not for others. In fact, 98% of all diets for weight loss fail. Of the people who lose weight, they will have regained as much or more than the weight they lost within three years.

I have studied more than 100 dietary theories, many with their creator in nutrition school, and understand their message and application. But where I feel the industry fails is that it does not teach how these diets relate to *you*. One person's food is another person's poison. One person may lose weight on pasta, while another may feel bloated, gassy and gain weight. What if you picked the wrong diet? The poisonous one? The one that saps your energy and causes all sorts of physical, mental and emotional issues?

There are certain dietary theories that recognize people's biological differences and recommend eating differently for different body types. The Blood Type diet, for instance, presents four diets based on the four blood types. The Ayurveda tradition provides different dietary and lifestyle guidelines based on your constitution or body type (dosha): Vata (winter dosha), Kapha (spring dosha) and Pitta (summer dosha). Traditional Chinese Medicine provides guidelines based on the five Elements, or energy fields, present in nature and in the human body in varying proportions: Wood, Fire, Earth, Metal (or Air) and Water.

So where does that leave you? With a great adventure ahead of you to discover what your body needs and what you want out of life. You are a unique individual, with your likes and dislikes, unique strengths, core values, dress code, and many more characteristics. What energizes you and motivates you differs from what energizes and motivates others. Can you think of an incentive announced by your employer or group leader to motivate your team to meet an aggressive deadline which was not much of a motivator for you? Maybe you were promised a spot bonus, but what you really wanted was a paid day off to make up for the lost time with your family or a weekend trip with your spouse?

Likewise, what wears you down and stresses you out may not affect someone else's well-being much at all. Skipping lunch as a result of a meeting running several hours late (sound familiar?) is fine for some people, but it was always unbearable for me. I felt like I was turning into an angry monster. From person to person, our threshold to various stress factors varies wildly. Discovering yours is part of this adventure.

Understanding what affects your digestion, your immune system and your sleep positively or negatively is an iterative process of self-reflection and observation. The answers lie in food and non-food related forms of nourishment.

You're not going to be left alone guessing, though. Your body and mind know what they need and tell you all the time. The voice of your body comes through food cravings and emotions.

Therefore, to understand what your body needs, you need to understand the secret language of cravings, comply with your body's demands, and acknowledge and fulfill your emotional needs. Your cravings for sweets may, for example, simply be cravings for energy because of a lack of sleep, or a craving for sweet and grounding root vegetables, which nourish your spleen, pancreas and stomach. It could in some instances be a sign, if you are vegetarian, that you are lacking protein. It could even be the need for a hug after a long stressful day, some sweetness in your life.

The answers are contained within yourself, your inner wisdom. Your body never makes mistakes.

While I do prescribe detailed nutritional guidelines in my private practice or in my group programs, my intention in this book is to give you guidelines that will enable you to experiment with foods for yourself. Which ones make you feel your best? Where can you find them on the road?

How do you integrate them into your day-to-day when you live on the go?

Bear in mind that you cannot change your diet without changing your sleep, exercise, and other areas of your life, because all aspects of your bio-individual regimen, or 'nourishment menu', are connected. However, if you implement the GDN blueprint, you may experience the following side effects: skyrocketing energy levels, deep sleep, weight loss, better skin and hair, improved digestion, less sickness, a happier mind, better flow of creative juices, faster thinking, upbeat mood and a fitter overall self.

What would I do if I had two more hours of high energy in the day?

_____
_____
_____
_____
_____
_____
_____
_____
_____
_____

If I did not feel sleepy, anxious, angry, tired, sore, heavy, or lethargic, what would it enable me to do and where would my career be?

_____
_____
_____
_____
_____
_____
_____
_____
_____

How will feeling my best affect others around me (loved ones, acquaintances, the wider world) and how will it affect other areas of my life?

_____

_____

_____

_____

_____

_____

_____

_____

_____

_____

_____

_____

_____

_____

_____

_____

Goal-directed nutrition will help you eat and take care of yourself to meet your career goals, even in the high-stress and fast-paced environment of Corporate America and the drain of business travel. I ask you to trust the process, experiment with food, and try establishing a self-care routine that will help you reclaim your health, increase your energy levels and reduce stress.

Now, pause for a moment to reflect on the story so far. The key to success in your professional career is not to work harder. You cannot force success with more overtime. The brilliant idea that will set you apart in the marketplace will likely not come out of an exhausted mind working round the clock on a client presentation deck, nor getting off a red-eye flight sleep-deprived. The key to career success is to feed your body with the most nutritious foods available, picked strategically, and to carve out time to renew yourself.

Physical beauty or attraction is earned, not bought at the beauty parlor. The attractive person attracts success at work, gets promoted, is staffed on the best projects, works with the best team members, is hired by the best clients, and sought after by the best leaders and mentors in the company. Can you think of a person at work who makes you feel miserable? What about someone who makes you feel amazing, someone you look up to and who motivates you to shine and give your best? Can you notice which of the two is the happier, more attractive and healthier person?

Being healthy creates a ripple effect of fulfillment everywhere: at work, within relationships, for exercise performance, spiritual connectedness, and financial health to name a few. On the contrary, suffering from poor health translates into continuous struggle in several areas.

Consultants, busy professionals and business travelers are flexible, highly adaptable, quick-learning and adventurous. Use these skills to change your dietary and lifestyle routine and unleash your superpowers.

PART II
GOAL-DIRECTED NUTRITION

5.
MILESTONE 1:
EAT FOR ENERGY AND
ATTRACTIVENESS

Eat to maintain high and continuous levels of energy throughout the day, without experiencing energy crashes, without feeling hungry, without experiencing digestive discomfort or gaining weight. Eat to feel attractive and charismatic, and walk the world with confidence and assurance. Eat for emotional stability, to feel a sense of belonging and inclusiveness, and to feel love(d).

I love eating. I love good food. I've traveled the world to learn how to cook local cuisines, taken classes in culinary schools on the American continent, in Europe and in Asia, and practiced with local chefs as well as local families. I've toured countries in search of the most authentic fare. I've driven two hours to get a taste of fresh goats' cheese on a farm or eat the perfect oyster. For the past nine years, I've saved the money I make teaching a 7.00am Monday morning indoor cycling class so that every six months I can cash it in and go eat a romantic dinner with my love in one of NYC's most exclusive restaurants, experiencing a half-day culinary extravaganza paired with the very best wines and liquors. The anticipation build-up is as exciting as the experience itself and it gets me super-motivated on the spin bike! I create recipes, organize gourmet dinners at my home and have written three cookbooks in support of my Gourmet Detox programs.

Rest assured. My intention is to keep the pleasure of eating very much alive here! But I deeply believe that we cannot eat the same way on our busy stressful days and on our relaxing days off. Party food gets in the way of us feeling our very best and being able to make our greatest impact in the world.

As discussed in the previous chapter, stress impairs digestion and elimination. Maintaining a healthy digestive and elimination system is essential to feeding success because of better fuel absorption, more energy, a lot less tiredness and sickness. Therefore, foods you eat on a busy work or travel day must be simple and easy to digest. At the same time, they must be extremely micro-nutrient-dense. When flying on commercial aircrafts especially, the lower pressure conditions and associated reduced oxygen levels in the cabins are similar to what mountain climbers experience. Would you eat filet mignon, a turkey sandwich with mayo or a bowl of pasta trekking your way up Mount Washington (about 6,000 feet)? Would you drink a cocktail or a glass of wine then? The digestive system becomes sluggish and absorbs fewer nutrients. At altitude, you experience more gas, bloating and overall digestive discomfort eating fatty foods and large meals, and the flavor of the food becomes bland, reducing the pleasure of eating.

Just as for athletes, your digestive system is your ultimate engine for high mental and physical performance. In this chapter, the fundamental ideas around improving digestion are that:

1. You choose the highest quality whole foods available, filled with life force;

2. You chose the simplest and lightest preparation or cooking method for this food;

3. You limit your intake of hard-to-digest foods even if they are high quality wholesome foods;

4. You steer clear of micro-nutrient-poor foods in order to not waste your limited digestive power (or your short meal break!) eating less important foods;

5. You try to create the best environment possible to enjoy eating your food, which will increase the rate of nutrient absorption by your body and your sense of joy;

6. You eat just the amount you need to feel your best and avoid over-eating. You do not eat for any other reason than fulfilling true hunger.

7. If you do this consistently, your life will transform in ways beyond your wildest dreams.

1.1:
EAT MORE FOODS WITH LIFE FORCE, WHOLE FOODS AND SUPERFOODS ON A DAILY BASIS.

Foods that are alive have life force. These include raw foods, unpasteurized foods, and fermented foods. Their nutrients are intact and have not been destroyed by processing.

Whole foods are foods that are close to their original and natural state or have only been minimally processed or cooked. A whole food was not man- or factory-made, but grew or was raised naturally. An orange is a whole food. Orange juice freshly pressed by you, less so. And commercial orange juice is not a whole food at all. Whole wheat is a whole food, because the grain contains all parts (the bran, germ, and endosperm). However, bread is made with flour, which is processed and not a whole food. A steak from a grass-fed pastured cow is wholesome, unlike a steak from a conventionally raised cow on grain, or cured meat, which is highly processed.

Superfoods have very high levels of nutrients, often off the charts with certain vitamins and minerals. They are nature's body boosters.

The most nutrient-dense whole foods and superfoods are plants. Therefore, the first rule is to make sure plants are the star of your meals, the centerpiece of your plate. The more micro-nutrients you eat for a given amount of calories, the easier the digestion process and the more energy you generate. Plus, your waist line may shrink down to its normal size. (Bonus!)

Next is a detailed prescription of 11 foods you should eat every day whether at home or on the road. They will provide the best information to your body, and increase and sustain your energy levels.

THE 'EAT MORE OF THAT' CHECKLIST

	Did you eat your share of wholesome, living foods today?	Minimum Daily Serving (see below for serving sizes)
1	Water	Half your ideal body weight
2	Dark leafy greens	2-3
3	Marine algae and freshwater algae	1
4	Spices and herbs	Unlimited daily
5	Superfoods	Unlimited daily
6	Sweet vegetables	1
7	Essential fats	1
8	Immune-boosting mushrooms, onions, garlic, and berries	2-3
9	Whole grains	1
10	Beans and lentils	1
11	Fermented foods, probiotics and digestive enzymes	1

The prescription serving for each food is the minimum amount of that food to be consumed. After a while, your body will crave these foods a lot and you'll find yourself eating more of them.

TO CALCULATE YOUR IDEAL WEIGHT & WATER INTAKE:

For women: Take number 100 for the first 5 feet of your height and add number 5 for every additional inch. Consider +/-10% depending on your body frame.

- *Example: I am 5'4", which equates to 100 + (5 x 4) = 120 lbs, +/-10% means 108 lbs to 132 lbs. I happen to weigh 128 lbs.*

- *Therefore, I would need about 64 oz of water daily (not counting the extra needed for exercise or compensating for caffeine and alcohol consumption).*

For men: Take number 106 for the first 5 feet of your height and add number 6 for every additional inch. Also consider +/-10% depending on your body frame.

- *If you are 5'8", this equates to 106 + (6 x 8) = 154 lbs, +/-10% means 139 lbs to 169 lbs.*

- *You would need about 77 oz of water daily.*

Note that serving sizes vary depending on the type of food you eat and how you prepare it:

- 1 serving of greens and vegetables is equal to 2 cups green lettuce, or 1 cup of raw, cooked or juiced vegetables.

- 1 serving of fruit is equal to 1 small sized fruit, ½ cup chopped fruit or ¼ cup dried fruit.

- 1 serving of legumes is equal to ½ cup cooked beans or lentils.

- 1 serving of animal protein or dairy is equal to 1 oz of cheese, 1 egg, a small yogurt, a deck of cards sized piece of chicken, meat, or fish.

- 1 serving of whole grains is equal to ½ cup cooked grains.

- 1 serving of essential fats is equal to ½ an avocado, 10 nuts, 1-2 tbsp of good quality oil.

- 1 serving of superfoods, including algae, is equal to 1 tsp to 1 tbsp depending on the superfood and your experience with it. The first time taking it, your dose will be lower.

Below is a description of each food, its benefits and how to integrate it into your diet.

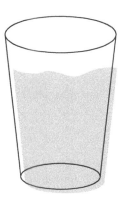

Prescription 1: Drink water. Drink half your ideal body weight of water throughout the day. More if you exercise. Drink two additional glasses of water for every glass of alcohol or caffeinated beverage consumed.

Description: Drink clean filtered tap water or bottled water (although there is a risk of leached chemicals from the plastic bottle). In our overly populated and industrialized world, water quality (and availability) is a big issue and an enabler to the spread of disease. One concern is that, although the authorities are doing their best to test and treat water, pesticides, heavy metals and other chemical contaminants like nitrates, arsenic and lead, as well as human and animal waste and microbes can still infiltrate a water supply. Out-of-date plumbing also poses health threats. (I should know! I live in a house over 100 years old). Finally, the water treatment in itself is a concern: chlorine and fluoride are poisons and, in the case of thyroid disease, exposure to both invariably makes my thyroid enlarge or throb.

Benefits: Did you know that experiencing poor digestion, sluggish thinking, skin breakouts, headaches, bad breath and general fatigue may be a sign of dehydration? Drinking adequate amounts of water keeps you energized. Your entire system shuts down when you are dehydrated so the first sign of dehydration is fatigue. Water is also an elixir of youth, it can clear dark circles, blemishes, and make you look years younger.

How to integrate it into your diet: Drink a full glass of water or lemon water first thing in the morning when you wake up to flush out the toxins from the previous day and to energize you. This will prepare your digestive system for better food absorption. I recommend you drink half your ideal body weight throughout the day, possibly more if you work in an air-conditioned office and travel in airplanes a lot. If you weigh 130 lbs, you'd need 65 oz of water. Drink half your water intake in the morning and the other half before 5.00pm. Drinking too close to bed time would lead to interrupted sleep at night. Try to drink a glass an hour. A good tip for when you're starting out is to set your alarm clock hourly to help you remember and start forming a habit.

Drink two additional glasses of water for every caffeinated or alcoholic beverage to offset the dehydration and stress caused on your system. When exercising, hydrate more with water. While it all depends on how much you sweat, a good rule of thumb for high intensity exercise such as a 60-minute indoor cycling class is 40 oz of water over the time period before, during and after the class.

Studies indicate that 80% of Americans are chronically dehydrated. I believe it! I noticed that my co-workers did not drink water in the office or on our business trips. They either did not drink anything between meals or they primarily drank soda, sugary vitamin water, sports drinks, coffee or green tea. Even at breakfast, I did not see any water on their desk but a 'pick-me up' hot beverage (ever seen those long Starbucks or Dunkin' Donuts wait lines in the morning?) At lunch at the cafeteria or out at restaurants and delis, it was a Snapple or another sweet drink. Then dinner was beer, wine and cocktails. In fact, most of them did not like the taste of water. If that's the case for you, I recommend you jazz up your water with a squeeze of lemon or orange, a slice of cucumber, or a teaspoon of crushed berries. Avoid commercial flavored water filled with chemicals.

I travel with my own stainless steel water bottle everywhere and refill it with filtered tap water in restaurants or coffee shops. Beware of water on airplanes. Years after the Environmental Protection Administration (EPA) finalized a consent decree with 24 US airlines failing drinking water tests, the quality of water is still precarious in 2014, showing coliform and E. coli present in major and smaller airlines alike. Now, what water do you think they use to brew your coffee on an airplane? Only disinfection will kill bacteria. Boiling water is not enough. Just sayin'...

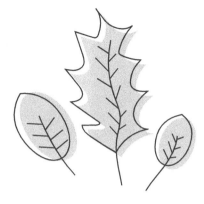

Prescription 2: Eat two to three servings a day of dark leafy greens and cruciferous vegetables.

Description: Dark leafy greens include plants like kale, chard, collard greens, dandelion, romaine lettuce and any other vibrantly green lettuce leaf, broccoli rabe, Chinese cabbage, spinach, and so on. The cruciferous vegetables, some of which are leafy, are plants from the cabbage family like broccoli, cauliflower, kale, bok choy, Brussels sprouts and all types of cabbage. Special mention to sprouts coming out in the spring, which are jam-packed with nutrition and vitality and come in different varieties like alfalfa, mung bean, lentil, radish, clover, sunflower, and broccoli sprouts.

Benefits: Dark leafy greens and sprouts are the most nutrient-dense, anti-inflammatory and detoxifying foods on the planet, along with algae. They are, thus, the most important foods you can eat to feed success. Sadly, they are also the most lacking foods from our modern diets. How many servings a day do you get? The greens are packed with vitamins A, C and E, minerals such as calcium, magnesium and iron, chlorophyll and fiber. They are voluminous and light at the same time, contributing to a feeling of satiety without a feeling of heaviness. Energetically, they foster a subtle, flexible and uplifting energy and help fight depression. The sprouts specifically make you feel very alive! Physically, they support the circulatory and respiratory system, clear congestion, and cleanse the liver, gallbladder, kidneys and blood. They also clear the skin, build internal gut flora and contain powerful anti-cancer compounds.

How to integrate them into your diet: The greens should be the star of your plate. Your meals should be built around them. What I love the most about land-based and aquatic greens is how quick they are to prepare. You can be ready to eat them raw or cooked in under five minutes. For the time-pressed professional, they are a godsend.

Each green requires a different preparation to enhance its flavor and increase its digestibility. Greens like kale require massaging before being eaten raw, but this isn't necessary for spinach. Most greens do well water sautéed, quickly boiled, stir-fried, and even grilled. Steaming however is not the best, making greens extra bitter. So buy a fresh vibrant green and search for how best to prepare it. A great cookbook covering the topic is *Greens Glorious Greens* by Johanna Albi and Catherine Walthers. You can also download the Feeding Success meal plans for recipe ideas from my website.

Sprouts can be added to salads and on top of any dish (soup, stir-fries, omelets, etc.) and inside wraps for a fresh crunchy taste. Younger sprouts are easier to digest.

When dining out, scan the menu for dishes including leafy greens and order a couple. They are usually found in the appetizer and side dish sections.

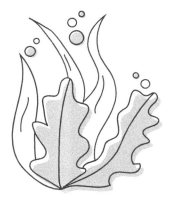

Prescription 3: Eat one serving of marine or freshwater algae daily.

Description: Algae are the aquatic kind of leafy greens. Algae are the earliest and oldest form of life on the planet. They have been around for billions of years! There are two kinds of algae: marine (also called sea vegetables or seaweed) and freshwater. The most common seaweeds include hijiki, kombu, wakame, arame, nori, dulse, sea palm and agar agar (Japanese names). Freshwater algae include the green algae chlorella, and the blue-green algae spirulina, aphanizomenon and other freshwater and marine phytoplankton.

Benefits: The longevity of algae speaks volumes about their amazing ability to regenerate and inspire life. Because of their iodine, trace elements and mineral content, algae were instrumental in my personal healing. Algae are extremely high in chlorophyll, beta-carotene and minerals (iron, zinc, calcium, potassium) and several vitamins (A, B1, B2, B3, B6 and B12, C, D, and E). They also contain all eight essential amino acids making them a great source of protein. Algae have antibacterial, antifungal and antiviral compounds. For this reason, they help build the good bacteria in the gut and support the strengthening of the digestive and immune systems.

Further, they are used in Japan in connection with cancer therapy treatment as they have been proven effective in slowing the growth of cancer cells in experiments. They have also proven useful to break down or cleanse the body of toxins, heavy metals, trans fat and other harmful chemicals. Given the frequent flyer's exposure to toxins and radiation, as well as high consumption of fried foods, adding algae to your diet is essential.

How to integrate them into your diet: Algae are an acquired taste for people who have not been brought up eating them. I was introduced to them when I studied the macrobiotic diet, native of Japan. You can find marine algae in all Japanese restaurants. Look for appetizers made of seaweed like three-color seaweed salad, miso soup with wakame seaweed, kukiwakame (marinated wakame seaweed), oshitashi (steamed greens like spinach with kombu seaweed sauce), hijiki sautéed with carrots, and sushi rolls made with nori seaweed.

There also exist seaweed snacks that you can eat on the go. At home, I cook my beans and whole grains with one inch piece of kombu and use agar agar instead of jello in my desserts.

Chlorella, spirulina and aphanizomenon can be found in powder forms and added in your green smoothies. You can also boost your orange juice or grapefruit juice in the morning with a teaspoon of spirulina powder for instance.

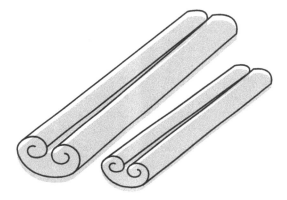

Prescription 4: Consume an unlimited amount of any of the world's most powerful spices and herbs daily.

Description: When you think of the healthiest foods on Earth, do spices come to mind? The truth is that spices are some of the top superfoods you can consume and should be a part of everyone's diet. Spices occupy eight of the top ten places on the ORAC scale (Oxygen Radical Absorbance Capacity) Basically, the ORAC scale ranks different foods according to the amount of antioxidants found therein. To be fair, this rating system is based on 100g of the food being analyzed. It's a lot easier to eat 100g of blueberries (ORAC placing 4,669) than of cardamom, but you get the point! Make sure you eat plenty of these super spices: turmeric, cloves, ginger, nutmeg (except for pregnant women), cinnamon, cardamom, vanilla bean and black pepper.

Herbs are aromatic and nutritious in equal measure. I attended a lecture given by raw-food guru David Wolfe in nutrition school where he mentioned that there were about 800 herbs discovered and inventoried for their medicinal purposes and many more hundreds waiting to be found! Popular fresh (or dried) herbs that you can start using daily include basil, cilantro, dill, mint, lavender, parsley, sage, oregano, thyme, rosemary, tarragon, chervil, chives, and bay laurel.

Benefits of spices: Spices are anti-inflammatory, antiviral, antibacterial, anti-carcinogenic, antiseptic, and antifungal. Depending on the spice, they help treat insomnia, tackle diabetes by moderating insulin levels, reduce serum cholesterol, improve IBS and gastrointestinal distress, treat candida and other bacterial infections, support brain health, prevent Alzheimer's Disease, cleanse the liver, act as painkillers, treat inflammatory conditions (arthritis), help prevent cancer, combat anxiety and depression, reduce symptoms of asthma and more. You get so much nourishment in just a teaspoon and your meals come to life with flavor.

Benefits of herbs: Herbs contain essential oils (some containing omega-3 oils), chlorophyll, vitamins A, B2, C and K, folic acid, minerals like iron, manganese and calcium and flavonoids and pigments, which have anti-cancer properties. Some of the effects of fresh herbs that I welcome as a busy professional are: they assist with digestion and help relax the intestinal lining; they have a detoxifying effect, especially parsley; and they're natural deodorizers. (Always nice to present fresh in front of a client!)

How to integrate them into your diet: You can add spices and herbs to your food upon serving or during the cooking process.

All the traditional cuisines of the world include spices, herbs, and other condiments that are specific to their culture because of their therapeutic properties and flavors. The French use garlic, dried or fresh herbs like sage, thyme, basil and rosemary. Chinese food often uses cloves, cinnamon and fennel seeds. Mediterranean cuisines typically use lemon with cumin, parsley, and oregano. The Indian subcontinent uses a wide variety of spices depending on the region, the most common of which are turmeric, coriander (or fresh cilantro), cumin, ginger and chili. Cuisines of Central and Latin America use different types of chilies, cactus leaves, cilantro, cumin, garlic and oregano. The southern US cuisine uses cayenne pepper, mustard seeds and paprika. Look for curry dishes. Curries are spice blends, but are not always hot. French curry, for instance, is very mild and does not include hot pepper. It tastes different from Indian, Thai and Jamaican curries, which are much hotter.

I recommend you vary your cooking style and experiment with spices and herbs. When dining out, try a variety of restaurants and look for the dishes that include health-promoting spices and condiments. You can also ask for extra herbs or spices in your food.

EMMA'S STORY

Personally, I travel with a little pouch of organic turmeric and cinnamon that I sprinkle on my food or in my morning tea (works on coffee too!) I also made a vanilla chai spice blend at home that I use as a digestive and to help me sleep at night. I sprinkle it on yogurt or oatmeal at the hotel and mix it with water or nut milk before bedtime.

I also carry turmeric pills that I eat after breakfast, lunch and dinner on the road. Turmeric is known to enhance digestion, reduce gas, bloating and acid reflux. It is also contains powerful antioxidant and anti-cancer compounds. I also travel with ginger teabags to support digestion, guard myself against colds and flu, reduce inflammation and combat motion sickness and with moringa leaf tea bags to boost my immune system.

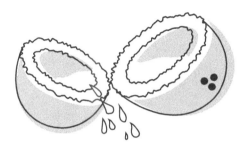

Prescription 5: Supplement your daily diet with a variety of superfoods.

Description: Superfoods are foods that have off-the-chart levels of nutrients in many categories. They must be eaten raw. Examples of recently popularized superfoods are: bee pollen, royal jelly, maca, cacao, coconut, aloe vera, hemp seeds, super berries like acai, camu camu, goji and Incan berries, and algae, mentioned above.

Benefits: Describing the benefits of each superfood named above would be the subject of a book in itself. In fact, I would recommend David Wolfe's excellent book *Superfoods* to get a detailed description of the world's top 10 superfoods. In a nutshell, consider these foods the most nutrient-dense or, otherwise said, those with the highest amount of nutrients per calorie. They are the ultimate health-boosters, containing super-concentrated levels of micro-nutrients, which can improve your overall health, by enhancing the function of multiple organs and systems in your body. You get a lot of bang for your nutrition buck without expanding your waist line. To quote David: "Superfoods are both a food and a medicine".

How to integrate them into your diet: When planning your meals and snacks, try to integrate superfoods as supplementation. They can easily be added to smoothies (super berries powder, aloe vera gel, bee pollen, homemade coconut milk) or used as snacks (raw cacao nibs, hemp seeds, coconut flakes). You can also top your 'regular' food with superfoods. For example, I sprinkle cacao nibs on top of my guacamole to give it a native Mayan flair and I blend hemp seeds in my salad dressing for added protein and omega-3 fatty acids.

In appendix 2, you'll find the superfood trail mix I make at home. I always take this with me on the road to have for or with breakfast, as a mid-afternoon snack, or in place of an in-flight dinner. Super delicious and nutritious!

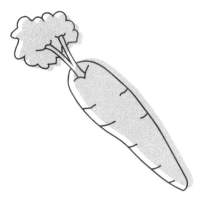

Prescription 6: Eat one serving a day of sweet vegetables.

Description: These include squash, carrots, turnips, parsnips, beets, yams, potatoes, sweet potatoes and the like. Surprisingly, sweet vegetables may not all taste sweet, even though they help satisfy your sweet cravings. Examples include radishes, onions, daikon, green cabbage and burdock root.

Benefits: A major benefit is that sweet vegetables satisfy a sweet tooth without compromising health like candy would! In fact, proactively including them in your meal will likely prevent the mid-afternoon sugar craving. Sweet vegetables soothe the internal organs such as the spleen, pancreas and stomach. Because many are root vegetables, they help us feel grounded, while processed sugar makes us feel high and spacey. Orange sweet vegetables are rich in vitamins C, A and beta-carotene. They assist in cancer prevention, promote eye health, delay cognitive aging and protect the skin against sun damage.

How to integrate them into your diet: Look for sweet vegetables in raw or cooked form at the salad bar and add them to your salad. You can also find them as a side on restaurant menus. Sweet potatoes, beets and turnips are particularly common in the fall. Carrots make excellent snacks by themselves or dipped in guacamole or hummus. Red radishes, daikon and green cabbage also help break down animal fats, which is why daikon is usually served in Japanese restaurant with sushi and sashimi.

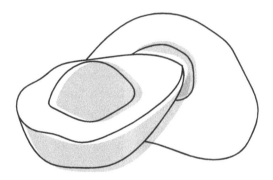

Prescription 7: Eat one serving a day of healthy fats.

Description: All fats are not created equal and foods containing fats usually contain more than one type. With that said, my general recommendation to you is to eat fats in their wholesome form as much as possible, and reduce processed and harmful fat intake.

Eat more monounsaturated fat such as olives and cold pressed olive oil, avocado, nuts (cashews, peanuts, almonds) and nut butters. These fats are whole foods (with the exception of olive oil, which is processed from the olive, so choose a high quality, unrefined, cold pressed oil in a dark glass bottle with an expiry date). These wholesome fatty foods also contain more nutrients and enzymes, which assist in the digestion of fats (lipase) and are also good protein sources.

Polyunsaturated fats from vegetable oils like safflower, sunflower, cottonseed, legumes (including soybean), and fatty fishes like salmon are also good choices. But stay clear of canola oil which is almost always GMO and highly processed.

When it comes to saturated fats, stick to enjoying the saturated fat from the coconut and the cacao bean. These are superfoods that contain incredible amounts of micro-nutrients. Otherwise, eat very limited amounts of saturated fats from animal products and make sure that you purchase high quality foods. Better options include whole-fat dairy products, full-fat yogurt, and grass-fed in-pasture hormone-free red meat and poultry (Poultry skin also contains polyunsaturated fat). I'd recommend limiting your intake of these fats during your high power days Monday-Thursday as they are harder to digest and might slow you down, make you feel tired and give you indigestion. Instead, enjoy them when you are less busy and not traveling.

Avoid all trans fat such as margarines, vegetable shortening, partially hydrogenated vegetable oil, deep fried chips/foods as it increases levels of LDL (bad cholesterol) as well as contributing to lowering your levels of good cholesterol (HDL). Even if a label indicates 'zero trans fat', bear in mind the food may still contain 0.5g of trans fat, the legal tolerance for foods to qualify as 'zero trans fat'. Read the ingredients carefully and if you see any of the ingredients listed at the beginning of this paragraph, do not eat! If you eat chips, fries, commercial baked goods and other processed foods during the day, for example, you could end up with 1.5g of trans fat or more in your system. And even though New York City banned trans fat in restaurants in 2008, fries are still fries; eating even a small amount can be harmful, slowly killing you!

Benefits: The benefits of fats depend on which fat you eat. Unrefined whole foods (avocado, nuts, fatty fish, coconut, olives) promote general health, soothe your nervous system, and power your brain and your body. Part of the reason why nuts and seeds are an excellent addition to the busy professional's diet is that they contain a high concentration of energy. However, they should be eaten in moderation (10 nuts in one serving) because they can create anxiety and nervousness if eaten in excess, according to Steve Gagné in his book *Food Energetics.*

How to integrate them into your diet: Remember, the presence of fat is necessary to absorb the fat-soluble vitamins (A, D, E and K), so they should be integrated into your diet, though carefully. The most important aspect is to control your intake of fat both from a source and a quantity standpoint. For this reason, ask for your food to be prepared with little or no fat, and then add it in yourself. Ask for your spinach to be water sautéed and your broccoli to be steamed. Ask the waiter to bring a side of olive oil and use your spoon to measure out one tablespoon. Ask for salad dressing to be served on the side. Remember not to duplicate your source of fat. If you have salmon, avocado, nuts and olive oil in the same meal, you're eating too much fat, burdening your digestive system, and slowing you down. (Don't forget we're trying to free up your energy!)

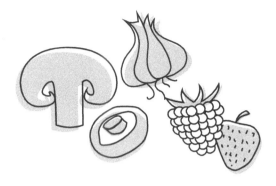

Prescription 8: Eat two to three servings a day of any of these other immune-boosting foods from the allium family, mushrooms, berries and fruit.

Description: All the foods discussed thus far are immune-boosting, but there are a few more that need special acknowledgement: the white vegetables in the allium family (onion, garlic, green onion, shallots, etc.) and mushrooms, as well as berries like blueberries, strawberries, blackberries and raspberries (when in season).

Benefits: The white vegetables are nature's pharmacy and a force to be reckoned with for business travelers exposed to all sorts of viruses and bacteria traveling for work. White veggies help lower LDL cholesterol, lower blood pressure and boost your immunity. Garlic and onions have antiviral and antibacterial phytochemicals. They contain powerful flavonoid antioxidants like quercetin, and help prevent inflammation. Together with a dose of ginger, they can help protect you against the winter cold and boost your defenses on a business trip. Mushrooms are fungi and have powerful anti-cancer properties, limiting tumor growth. In his book *Super Immunity*, Dr. Joel Fuhrman describes mushrooms (and other foods) as anti-angiogenic. He explains that they contain nutrients that inhibit angiogenesis, meaning they prevent tumors from growing. In fact, he cites a Chinese study, which showed that women who ate 10g of mushrooms daily saw a decrease in their risk of breast cancer by 64%. They also prevent fat cells from expanding, stop inflammation and inhibit the development of cancer. Equally powerful, berries are highly immune-boosting. Along with other red vegetables and fruit, berries are loaded with powerful, healthy antioxidants, which soak up damaging free radicals. They may do everything from fight heart disease and prostate cancer to decrease the risk for stroke and macular degeneration, which is the leading cause of blindness in people aged 60 and over.

How to integrate them into your diet: Eat berries at breakfast or as a snack, and include raw garlic and onions to your salad or gently sautée them to give flavor to your cooked foods. There is a wide range of mushrooms to enjoy and they come in dried or fresh form. Simply rehydrate the dried mushrooms in a little water before use. Portobello and button mushrooms are found on most American restaurant menus and Asian restaurants present a larger variety such as oyster, shiitake, maitake and reishi mushrooms. They also come as a supplement extract.

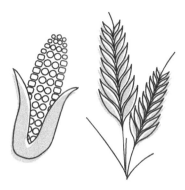

Prescription 9: Eat one serving a day of whole grains for long-lasting endurance.

Description: Whole grains have a bad reputation in the US. If you follow the fine print in nutrition news, you will know that several factors are to blame for the bad press. Namely, hidden sugar, excess processing, the use of genetically modified wheat, the addition of food additives in the bread, and over-consumption. Grains in their wholesome form are essential in human consumption and have been traditional in every diet around the world since agriculture was developed around 12,000 years ago.

Grains provide long-lasting energy for the body and are a great winter food, coming from the fall harvest season. Some grains are easier to digest than others. Glutinous grains such as wheat, couscous, bulgur and barley are hearty and more difficult to digest because the gluten makes these grains' consistency more glue-like. They also create more heat in the body, hence best suited for the winter months. Non-gluten grains include oats, quinoa, amaranth, millet, rice, corn and buckwheat (also called kasha if pre-roasted).

Benefits: Each whole grain has its own nutritional profile and story of growth in a different geographical location and climate. For this reason, the energetics of grains is all over the map, cooling and damp for the paddy rice, warm and damp for oats native of Scotland, Northern Europe and Germany, warm and dry for quinoa growing at altitude in the Andes mountains, hot and dry for buckwheat, which thrives in cold, damp and windy climates where the locals most need it to keep warm and strong like in Russia. Generally speaking, whole grains contain essential enzymes, iron, dietary fiber, vitamin E and B-complex vitamins making them an important foundation for anyone's diet.

How to integrate them into your diet: How much and what kind to eat depends on your bio-individuality. When feeding for success, quality over quantity matters. Avoid processed grains like white bread, and confectionary goods, which may make you feel lethargic, give you a headache and spike your blood sugar, leading to a sugar crash later. I recommend that the busy professional chooses sprouted and/or fermented breads for ease of digestion such as Ezekiel breads. Unless you have access to a bakery making the bread fresh that day, favor frozen breads which contain far fewer preservatives. Watch out for added sugar, white flour, enriched white flour, and so on. Traditionally, bread is made simply of flour, salt, water and sometimes yeast (but not always). There should be no molasses, syrup, or cane sugar. I also recommend eating the easier-to-digest gluten-free grains in their wholesome form during the power part of your week. Whole grains are a great compliment to vegetables in a dish, instead of saturated animal fat. For weight loss, typically I advise half a cup of grains per day (one serving), and for athletic development, one to one and a half cup per day (two or three servings).

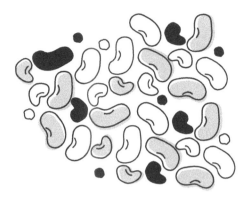

Prescription 10: Eat one serving a day of legumes (beans or lentils).

Description: Legumes are lentils, beans and peas. They come in many shapes and colors and are found in every single cuisine in the world. Lentils and the smaller beans like adzuki and mung beans are quicker to prepare and easier to digest while soybeans and chickpeas (or garbanzo beans) are the hardest to digest.

Benefits: Rich in folic acid, minerals such as iron, magnesium, potassium and soluble fiber, they are also a great source of low-fat protein and assist in lowering LDL cholesterol. They nourish your adrenal glands and kidneys. (Have you ever noticed the shape of a bean?) This can help restore your vital energy, including your libido. Beans also increase your endurance and level of satiety. The slow release of carbohydrates in the blood stream enables a consistent release of energy. Beans also help with normal bowel movement and regulate blood sugar. Several of my busy clients found that eating beans cured their sweet cravings and mid-afternoon bingeing if they ate legumes at lunchtime.

Beans are satisfying and have a calm and soothing energy.

How to integrate them into your diet: You can find beans in every restaurant out there. Pinto, black and kidney beans are more common in Latin American restaurant (chilies and burritos), chickpeas in Mediterranean cuisine (hummus, with couscous dishes). My favorite bean is the flageolet, praised in French cuisine and typically served with baby lamb dishes and my favorite lentils are the French lentils or *lentilles DuPuy.* Adzuki and soy beans are a staple of the Japanese macrobiotic diet, and Indian restaurants have all kinds of lentils dishes (green, red and black lentils) as well as chickpeas. To make your experience with beans more pleasant, eat small amounts (half a cup is a serving) and pair them with vegetables, rather than animal fat. There are also guidelines to follow if you prepare them at home to increase digestibility such as soaking them overnight and adding cumin or fennel seeds, kombu or kelp to the cooking water.

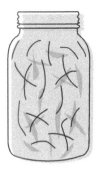

Prescription 11: Eat one serving a day (or more) or fermented foods, probiotics and enzymes.

Description: Fermented foods are the most alive of all foods. They are raw and contain living beneficial bacteria created by the fermentation process. Every culture has its fermented foods: yogurt (fermented milk), kimchi (Korean cuisine staple of fermented cabbage), sauerkraut (German staple of fermented cabbage), kombucha (fermented green tea from China back with the Chinese Tsin Dynasty), kefir (originating centuries ago in the Caucasus Mountains, now made with water, coconut water, or milk), and fermented fruit and vegetables in the Indian sub-continent and South East Asian countries, and mushrooms, yeast, olives, vinegar and wine on the European continent. Fermented beverages go as far back as 9,000 years ago according to a 2011 report from the United Nations' Food and Agriculture Organization.

Benefits: As we're about to discover in the coming chapters, one common root cause for many diseases is inflammation and bad bacteria taking over our body. Fermented foods provide us with probiotics and enzymes, which populate our gut and support our digestive system. Good gut bacteria help manufacture vitamins, digest food, boost the immune system, protect our nervous system, and so many other things. There are many more bacteria than there are cells in our body, respectively 100 trillion bacteria for 5 to 55 trillion cells (depending on the size of the human). Probiotics ensure the right kind of bacteria are fed. Interestingly, research reported in a *New York Times* article by Carl Zimmer on August 14th, 2014 stated: "Perhaps our menagerie of germs is also influencing our behavior in order to advance its own evolutionary success—giving us cravings for certain foods, for example."

I know this to be true! The more bad bacteria you have, the more bloated and mentally foggy you feel and the more sugar you crave, perpetuating the vicious circle. Has this not been your experience as well? Eating fermented foods, like sauerkraut, will help you address your sweet tooth, as fermented foods taste sweet to the body, yet feed the good bacteria with probiotics.

Fermented foods also provide you with enzymes. Enzymes are made of protein and are the catalyst for every chemical reaction in our body. Without adequate levels of enzymes, digestion is impaired, taxing your system even more.

How to integrate them into your diet: At home, eat three tablespoons of sauerkraut or kimchi with one of your meals or as a snack. You can also drink one kombucha a day, or enjoy a kefir drink for breakfast or as a snack. Supplementing with probiotics and enzymes may be a good idea too. When trying to populate your gut with good bacteria, it is best to take the probiotic supplements between meals rather than at meal time.

Otherwise, the probiotics will start digesting the food you're eating right at that time.

1.2
CROWD OUT THE ENERGY SAPPERS AND BAN WHAT CAUSES YOU HARM.

When you eat more of the good foods, you crowd out the hurtful foods naturally. Essentially, when you stay nourished, your cravings for junk food disappear. You'll have to trust me on that and give it a fair try! It does not take long. In fact, my clients experience this change within the first two weeks of our collaboration. The 'crowding out strategy' is more efficient than the usual calorie restriction or removal-only diet because it keeps you nourished.

Three-quarters typically experience drastic weight loss and an increase in energy right away, because the minute they stop hurting themselves, their body begins the mending process. Immediately.

The 11 foods listed below decrease your energy, increase your physical, mental and emotional stress, and increase your risk of disease. For this reason, I recommend steering clear of these foods on your big power days (and hopefully beyond, as some of these foods are not safe for humans!). If you eat meat, chicken, fish and other animal products on a regular basis, I ask that you limit your intake to no more than once or twice a week, preferably on your days off. If this is too hard, limit your intake to no more than once a day on your big days and select the highest quality available. If you are eating the 11 nutrient-dense foods daily, there won't be room in your stomach to eat much of the less nutritious or harmful foods.

Be prepared to skip a meal if only toxic food is available, like fasting on a flight. I'm dead serious! Remember your goals? I chose hunger over aging and sickness any day.

THE 'EAT LESS OR NONE OF THAT' CHECKLIST

Any allergies or food intolerance to consider first?	
1	Sugar
2	Chemicals and soft drinks
3	Alcohol
4	Coffee and caffeine
5	Table salt
6	Processed grains, baked goods, bread, pasta
7	Processed soy products
8	Dairy and whey protein
9	Low quality protein powder, milk and bars
10	Poor quality meat, too much or too little meat
11	Farm-raised fish and fish high in mercury

How strict you'll be in removing these foods depends on how fast you want to reach your goals as well as on your bio-individual tolerance for these foods and the effect they have on you.

Prescription 1: Check your body for food intolerance or allergies and remove allergens.

The biggest energy sapper is sickness. The second biggest? In my opinion, digestive stress. Digestion is already a huge energy demand on your body when your system is healthy, but when compromised it can suck the life out of you. If you experience headaches, nausea, fogginess, bloating, diarrhea, constipation, drops in energy, pain in your stomach, intestines, joints, back, or neck, you may be experiencing digestive stress and food toxicity. Digestive disorders can be severe like Celiac disease, Crohn's disease, Irritable Bowel Syndrome (IBS), Inflammatory Bowel Disease (IBD), gallstones, diverticulitis, or they can be more insidious like mild food allergies and sensitivities. Without the onset of a condition, these are tricky to test for.

You can find out whether you are sensitive to the typical allergens—wheat, gluten, corn, soy, dairy and sugar—by cutting them out of your diet for seven days and seeing how you feel, then adding them back one by one. More and more people are also intolerant to nuts and seafood. When you remove harmful foods from your diet, you start feeling better right away, less in pain and with increased energy and mental focus. By not eating the first two items on my list, sugar and chemicals, you can completely turn around your health and energy levels without having to remove or reduce your intake of the other nine. But if you do, you'll become an entirely new person in just a few months. Personally, I had to initially remove all 11 to heal Graves' disease, discover how powerful I was and dare taking my life to the next level. I reintroduced some of them in moderation, carefully experimenting when I was out of the woods. It was a very difficult and step-by-step learning process for me as no-one at the time really spoke about the relationship between auto-immune disorders, physical, mental and emotional stress, and diet and lifestyle. Here, I am giving you the recipe.

What foods am I allergic or sensitive to?

_____

_____

_____

Looking back at page 63, the foods I listed as giving me indigestion are also part of the 11 foods to crowd out. They are:

_____

_____

_____

_____

_____

After eating these foods I feel:

_____

_____

_____

_____

_____

_____

And this is how it affects my work day:

_____

_____

_____

_____

_____

_____

_____

Prescription 2: Crowd out the 11 foods that increase inflammation in your body and are hard on the digestive system.

Let's review them together. I hope the information below will convince you that these foods undermine your health and vitality, then feed your motivation to try to crowd them out.

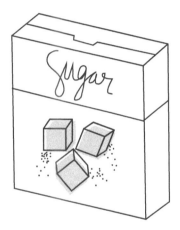

1. White (and brown) sugar. Sugar is without a doubt, along with chemical food additives, the highest cause of inflammation and heightened acidity in the body. Sugar creates a spike in blood sugar, followed by a spike in insulin, which converts sugar into fat raising your triglyceride levels. It also inhibits fat loss. Riding this rollercoaster over time leads to the development of insulin resistance and diabetes.

Sugar feeds bad bacteria, as well as cancer cells. Sugar saps your energy, as a sugar crash always follows the sugar high. It lowers immune function, causes migraines, obesity, bloating, PMS symptoms, stress and more.

Sugar is in so many things, for the great part without your awareness, including in savory (even salty) packaged foods, prepared meals, low-fat foods (the sugar makes up for the lack of flavor from the missing fat), sodas, sports drinks, and more. In the US, the average American consumes between 150 and 175 lbs of sugar a year! That's about half a cup every day. And if you've tried, you know that quitting is hard. Sugar is very addictive. "It is Americans' recreational drug", to quote Mark Hyman, founder and director of the Institute of Functional Medicine and author of *The Blood Sugar Solution*. According to him, it is the primary cause of diabesity.

Quit sugar and replace it with fresh fruits for an on-the-go snack or with gentle natural sweeteners like raw honey, real maple syrup, agave nectar, molasses, coconut and brown rice syrup, green leaf stevia (not the white processed extract or the drops), and date sugar.

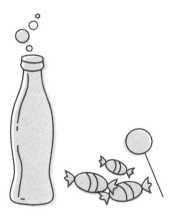

2. *Chemicals and soft drinks.* Chemicals are so damaging for your body and, let's be honest, there is no safe minimum level. What is even more worrisome is that your body is not equipped to digest them so, unless you detox, they remain stored in your fat cells (sometimes for decades) leading to serious health issues. In fact, the more exposed you are to chemicals and heavy metals, the more fat your body will manufacture to store these dangerous toxins away from your vital organs, making you fatter and increasing the likelihood of diseases.

Examples of such chemicals include high fructose corn syrup (HFCS), MSG (excitotoxin), artificial sweeteners, food coloring (red dye 40, yellow dye 5, and others), 'natural' flavors, fillers, preservatives, etc. These chemicals wreak havoc on your hormones, increasing ghrelin (the hunger hormone), lowering leptin (the satiety hormone), leading to insulin resistance, depleting your body of vitamins and minerals, and running down your immune system. Over 90 side-effects have been documented in the study of artificial sweeteners, aspartame being the worst of the worst. Colorings are synthetic chemicals derived from coal tar and can contain lead and arsenic. Preservatives such as EDTA have been linked to kidney failure and seizures. Benzene, a carcinogen, has been linked to leukemia and lymphomas. And phosphoric acid has been linked to osteoporosis, kidney stones and other diseases. Pesticides are also poisonous chemicals. If it kills a bug, do you honestly think it is safe for you? To stay current with the list of sprayed produce that receives the most and least chemicals, review the list produced by the Environmental Working Group posted on their website (ewg.org). As you'll read, EWG analyzes pesticide residue testing data from the US Department of Agriculture and Food and Drug Administration to come up with rankings for popular fresh produce items.

Below are the top 16 most-contaminated products. The lower the number, the more pesticides:

1. Apples

2. Strawberries

3. Grapes

4. Celery

5. Peaches

6. Spinach

7. Sweet bell peppers

8. Nectarines—imported

9. Cucumber

10. Cherry tomatoes

11. Snap peas—imported

12. Potatoes

13. Peppers

14. Blueberries—domestic

15. Lettuce

16. Kale or collard greens

When you eat organic foods, your body detoxifies chemicals and grows healthier. You biggest exposure to disease-causing pesticides and chemicals is through diet, followed by household cleaning products, detergents, hygiene and self-care items, then maybe your backyard. Take a wider look at your surroundings once you've eliminated chemicals from your diet. A resource to remove known or suspected carcinogens from your life and your home is *The Safe Shopper's Bible* by David Steinman and Samuel Epstein.

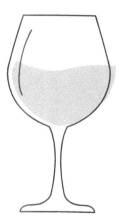

3. Alcohol. Alcohol is a toxic substance, even if you justify drinking your glass of red wine because of it provides you with healthy antioxidants! You're speaking to a woman who lived in Bordeaux for 10 years and has an uncle who makes the best Armagnac. Regardless, it still burdens the liver, which has to produce a special enzyme to break it down (ADHL) into acetic acid (vinegar, basically). A stressed liver negatively affects digestion, blood filtering, fat metabolism, and so many other functions that the liver is responsible for. Some people experience nasal congestion after drinking alcohol, caused by the inflammatory effect of the histamine produced by the body in response to alcohol. You experience congestion, excess mucus, possibly light flushing, the sum of which can negatively affect the quality of work and sleep. Have you ever noticed that your sleep is more interrupted or agitated after drinking alcohol? Have you noticed feeling hotter and sweatier?

Mentally, alcohol is a depressant. Hardly the effect we're after when feeding success! It is also an extreme yin food, whereby consuming it will lead to cravings for extreme yang foods like fatty foods (cheese, meat, salt, potato chips, etc).

Under the influence, all self-control goes out of the window. There is a lot of alcohol consumed on the road and at home in the life of the busy professional. "That glass or two really helped me unwind after work this evening", you tell yourself. What would happen if you decided not to drink at night during your big days? How would you unwind? Or better, how would you rearrange your day to not be wiped out by the end of it, and feeling the need for alcohol and chemicals to unwind or stay up late? These questions will be central to the subsequent chapters of the book.

I would recommend for now that you abstain from drinking alcohol during your power days (Monday to Thursday) to improve the quality of your sleep, to keep your mind alert and cheerful, and to prevent further dehydration, which makes you tired and slow. Above all, skip the drink on airplanes to prevent further dehydration. In social settings, consider drinking two glasses of still water for every alcoholic beverage.

4. Coffee and caffeine. The coffee bean is without question a very powerful one and has been used for medicinal purpose since it was discovered. There are pros and cons to drinking coffee and caffeine beverages, and your experience is bio-individual. The pros include increased focus and concentration, endurance and asthma relief for instance. The reason I recommend limiting or breaking the caffeine habit entirely is because it robs you of your awareness of how much natural energy you really have, as this is disguised by excessive consumption. It was never meant to be had daily, or even weekly. It was a digestive, for consumption after a big meal. Consuming caffeine because you are tired and need to boost your energy is the wrong reason to drink caffeine. Coffee is like a credit card. It creates an even greater energy debt. Eventually, after borrowing fake energy for too long, instead of addressing the root cause of your exhaustion upfront, the time comes for payback. If your debt is too great, you are in serious trouble, with your other health assets sinking into the pit one by one: your nervous, digestive, and endocrine systems to name a few. Coffee has been linked to adrenal exhaustion, ageing (of the skin and kidneys), cardiovascular problems, stress, emotional disturbances and mood swings. Coffee creates a spike in blood sugar, followed by a surge of insulin and later a sugar crash, similar to the consumption of sugar and alcohol.

Coffee and caffeine are also acidic and can create gastrointestinal problems (acid reflux, ulcers), female and male health problems. A female client found that drinking coffee was causing cysts in her breasts, which would disappear when she stopped her coffee intake. Other clients of mine saw their menopausal symptoms worsen with coffee, experienced infertility, and other problems. Caffeine inhibits the absorption of some nutrients and causes the urinary excretion of calcium, magnesium, potassium, iron, and trace minerals.

For all these reasons, because you want to know what it feels like to be your own natural best, I'd like you to get out of the coffee and caffeine *addiction*. If you want to keep drinking caffeinated beverages or coffee, even one cup a day, you'll rob yourself of that true feeling. Experiment for a few weeks. Reserve the use of coffee to strategic moments, not as a daily pick-me-up habit. Caffeinated tea, especially black tea, is also addictive. Opt for green or white tea in limited amounts, or herbal tea unlimited. Remember to drink two glasses of water after each intake of caffeine and to select organic teas and coffees to limit exposure to pesticides. Decaf coffee is even more toxic than regular coffee as the process of decaffeinating includes additional use of chemicals.

If you decide to stop, give yourself four or five days to get over the painful withdrawal phase. You'll soon feel an energy you did not know existed.

It is a great natural high accompanied by mental clarity and lightness. For more information about caffeine, read *Caffeine Blues: Wake Up to the Hidden Dangers of America's #1 Drug* by Stephen Cherniske.

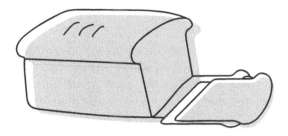

5. Processed grains, as in bread, pasta, baked goods, and commercial cereals. As discussed, compared to whole grains, processed grains do not provide adequate nutrition. They are a sub-quality food so look at it as a treat rather than nutrition. Learning how to read labels is the most important thing with processed grains. Watch out for undesirable food additives. Here are a few tips to keep in mind when evaluating the nutrition label and packaging of the cereal, bread, pasta or other pantry item you're buying:

- Avoid products with health claims.

- Avoid products that claim to be light, low-fat, reduced fat or fat-free, as they are loaded with sugar.

- In the ingredients list, avoid chemicals, preservatives, artificial flavors and colors.

- If you cannot pronounce it, don't eat it.

- The ingredients are listed in order of the largest to the smallest amounts. Brown rice should list brown rice. Ideally, bread should be made with unrefined flour, water, salt (and maybe yeast). Don't buy food with a long list of ingredients.

- Watch out for duplicate ingredients called differently. Sugar and fat have many names, which when totaled would equate to a larger proportion of these foods in the ingredient list. Most cereals are sugar bombs with cleverly designed packages and labels to trick the customer. Keep the sugar per serving amount under 7g.

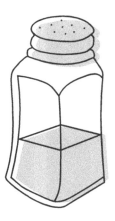

6. *Table salt.* Also called sodium chloride, salt is everywhere in today's packaged foods, even sweet foods, and does not have nutritional value. (The same is true of Kosher salt). It is linked to several issues, in addition to hypertension, which were listed in an research article published in the *Journal of Human Hypertension* in 2002. Paraphrasing the article, it can be said that salt led to a thickening of the arteries, growth of the left ventricle, and a negative impact on calcium and bone density especially in post-menopausal women. Salt also increases the number of strokes and cardiac failures and deteriorates kidney function. It controls the incidence of stomach cancer and has a negative impact on asthmatic patients. Salt also kills good bacteria (salt is antibacterial, hence its use to conserve foods); as we know, good bacteria are needed for a healthy immune system and preventing obesity. Salt also constipates, by removing water from your body. On the other hand, *eaten in moderation,* high quality, mineral-rich salts (like Himalayan rock salt, which contains over 80 minerals, or grey sea salt) are healthy and promote normal functioning of the human body.

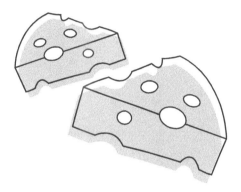

7. Dairy products. There is a lot of controversy over dairy. So you'll need to experiment and discover on your own whether dairy is good for your body or not. In nutrition school, I heard both sides of the story. It was the Weston A. Price Foundation, who lectured us on the pros of fresh raw milk, butter, cheese and cream, that captured all my attention. Growing up in France, I felt drawn to Sally Fallon Morell's speech, which justified the nutritive powers of butter and cheese... (My cheese platter!) Good quality (raw) dairy has an alkaline effect on the body, but raw milk is hardly available, or legal, to buy in many states. Note that hard aged cheeses are acidic and that the pasteurization process alters the protein molecule of milk, rendering it hard to digest and increasing inflammatory properties.

The reason dairy is on my don't-eat list is that it will likely increase the intensity of seasonal allergies, sinus congestion and inflammation, even ear infections, and make you less alert and efficient. Because it is inflammatory, I found that all of my clients suffering from joint and back pain benefited from quitting milk and cheese. When I eat cheese at night, I have a hard time breathing when I sleep; I feel congested the next morning and foggy. The real issue I think lies in the quality of dairy. Dairy cows in the US are fed GMO grains, hormones and antibiotics, none of which is very good for you. So during your power days, avoid dairy. Reserve it for days off and make sure it's very high quality product from grass-fed pastured cows when you do choose to consume it. Throughout the summer into the fall, you can find organic pastured butter in the stores. It has a creamy yellow color, smells wonderful and has a nutty flavor. Perfect for my Sunday morning *tartine* treat, but not for the busy weekdays, which start with a green smoothie.

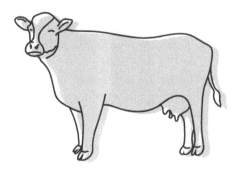

8. Conventionally raised animals and processed meats.
There is a growing awareness in the US and in the world of the environmental impact of the meat industry, as well as the harm caused by eating sick animals of any kind and low

quality processed meat. For humans, the connection these have to disease is especially prominently showing up as digestive and colon cancers. This is one reason why animals are on my 'eat less' list.

The other reason has to do with the effort involved in digesting meat. High-fat foods sit in the stomach for longer periods of time after consumption, requiring greater energy levels, which we are trying to free for other purposes than digestion.

In addition to eating less beef, the quality you chose to eat is paramount. A pastured cow is exposed to the sun and fed with grass, so it is a good source of omega-3 fatty acids, iron and B12. A conventionally raised cow on the other hand, which spends its life indoors, does not contain omega-3s but excess omega-6s, fat and hormones. They are frequently sick and inflamed as they are given GMO grains to eat, which they cannot digest. The energetics of grass-fed beef and suffering animals is vastly different. From a human health and performance standpoint, I recommend you abstain from eating meat until you can find the right quality. Ask the waiter at the restaurant if the cow is grass-fed and raised on pasture.

Energy-wise meat increases inflammation (heat) according to Ayurveda, TCM and food energetics, which worsens the inflammation created by stress and lack of sleep in the human body. Portion-wise, consume no more animal food (meat, chicken, or fish) than a deck-of-card-sized portion and preferably eat it on your days off, when your digestive system is more relaxed. Stay away from cured meats. If you were to indulge just as a one-off, be careful of the meat quality and the food additives included during processing. Choose nitrate-free products, with no added sugar, dairy or other fillers, and ensure you select products without casing. These guidelines apply to turkey, chicken and other animals. I would recommend you skip or eat less of those on your high power days for sure.

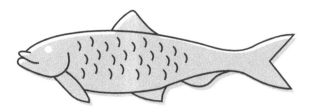

9. Farmed and larger predator fish. The problem with poor quality fish is the excess omega-6 fatty acids, which again are inflammatory, as well as the fish's exposure to mercury. One of my fellow management consulting directors was diagnosed with mercury poisoning, and since fish is the primary source of dietary mercury poisoning, this was the likely culprit. When on the road or in the office, she would chose fish over other animal protein several times a week, thinking it was the lighter, 'healthier' version. Do you ever chose fish thinking it is the healthier or less 'heavy' choice on the menu? Ayurvedic practitioner John Douillard, in his 'five safety rules for eating fish' communiqué, reported that a study showed: "20% of the fish at the sushi bar is over the mercury legal limit of 1 part per million [and] 184 samples of fish from lakes and streams around the US showed that half was over the limit and every single fish had mercury in it."

The bigger predators or scavenger fishes have the greatest levels of toxicity, namely mercury and PBS (from the plastic in the ocean). These fish include: shark, tuna, swordfish, sea bass, catfish and carp. Eating wild salmon swimming in very pure streams may be your safest bet, but no more than once, maybe twice a week according to John Douillard and other experts. If you exceed this amount, you will store mercury in your fat cells and brain since your brain is 45% fat… Personally, I stopped eating tuna years ago, in any shape or form, and limit my fish intake to no more than once a week. Generally, I choose the wild-caught salmon, trout or the fatter fishes which I've always loved (anchovies, herring, and sardines).

Steer clear of farmed fishes as they are also a health hazard. Fish can be sick, malnourished, and fed coloring and other harmful toxins in these environments. Try to find fish from a sustainable farm with good practices. (That means reading the labels and doing your research). I also try to avoid fish from polluted waters, which drastically reduces the options given the recent environmental catastrophes for fish coming from clean waters. I have bought more fish from fishermen at the local farmer's market and in the freezer section of my health food store, which has quality fish from a sustainable farm with good practices and ample space for the fish.

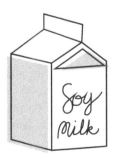

10. Processed soy products. Soy is another of controversial food. The research links it to cancer, but also cancer prevention for certain female cancers, namely breast and ovarian. I recommend you stay clear of highly processed soy products such as soy milk, soy cheese, fake meat and protein powder made of soy protein isolate, as well as soy ice cream. Even tofu should be eaten in limited amounts. On the contrary, I believe that non-GMO, organic and fermented soy products in small quantities like tempeh, shoyu and miso present health benefits due to the fermentation process. Edamame, young soy beans, are okay as well, but a little harder to digest than fermented soy products.

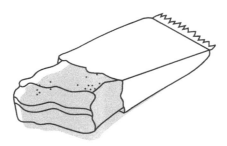

11. Poor quality protein powders, meal replacement drinks, protein bars and whey protein powders. These are convenient meal replacements for many busy professionals or business travelers if you can find high quality options. For this reason, I started to make my own formula in order to feed myself with the highest level of nutrition in a convenient way. My advice to you is to make sure that the type you use does not contain whey protein (the most processed form being whey isolate protein), soy isolate, sugar and artificial sugar, preservatives, flavoring, so-called 'natural' flavors and other food additives that will damage your health. Whey protein isolate is highly processed, using many chemicals that you do not want in your body. These chemicals denature the whey (which is a waste product from the cheese industry) to the point that the body has a hard time recognizing it as food. It contains bovine blood proteins, serum albumen, lactalbumin, dead white blood cells and hormonal residues including estrogen, and progesterone. This causes an immune response. Whey isolate is high in IGF-1 (insulin growth factor 1), which is a hormone that has been linked to cancer in some studies. It is highly inflammatory and some studies show increased risk of certain diseases including cancer, Parkinson's and Alzheimer's. Whey also causes an immune response when ingested, since the body sees it as a foreign invader (*The Lancet,* 1996). There are also links to diabetes according to the *New England Journal of Medicine,* 1992, and with multiple sclerosis as per the *Journal of Immunology,* 2001. This constantly stresses the immune system and can lead to auto-immune disorders.

I am convinced these chemicals were instrumental in the development of my auto-immune condition as I relied a lot on fitness nutrition supplements in my athletic life and for food-on-the go in my professional life, thinking (wrongly) that they were 'healthy' portable alternatives. Back then, no-one knew or questioned the industry. Since that time, however, there have been more consumer reports, independent food reviews and resources available and these have shed light on food safety like never before. These resources are particularly useful when considering replacements and supplements: WebMD (webMD.com), Green Med Info (greenmedinfo.com), NutritionFacts.org and the Food Babe Vani Hari (foodbabe.com). When your food starts making big news like this, and you get into reading it, it will change your food habits instantly. There are well-known protein drinks that you can find in gyms and stores alike that were found and reported in consumer reports to contain all four heavy metals (arsenic, cadmium, lead, and mercury). Now really... Do you want to eat that?

All it boils down to… Our body is naturally slightly alkaline, and continuously works to achieve homeostasis and maintain a pH level a little over 7.0. When the blood becomes overly acidic because of eating excessive amounts of the foods above, the body starts to leach more of the calcium stored in the bones into the blood (normally 2% of the body's calcium is stored in the blood) to re-establish the pH balance. You can see how an acidic diet may lead to osteoporosis. You can supplement calcium all you want, but it won't fix the problem, only worsen it by increasing calcium deposit throughout the body, in your joints, arteries and brain.

Inflammation is 'the silent killer'. So says *Time Magazine*. Indeed, inflammation is now believed to be the most common cause of diseases such as heart disease (inflammation of the arteries), Alzheimer's (inflammation of the brain), fibromyalgia (inflammation of the nervous system), arthritis (inflammation of the joints or the bones), eczema (inflammation of the skin), and even obesity (inflammation of the gut due to excess bad bacteria and infection). Inflammation is a normal reaction to injury or illness. It is not normal to have a body continuously inflamed without any way of turning off the inflammation.

Prescription 3: Avoid over-eating, especially protein.

Over-eating is taxing on the system. It lengthens the digestion process and creates lethargy. Not quite the vibe a busy professional is looking for. Most people need three to four hours to digest their food, but it can take several days to exit the system. Remember that prompt and healthy digestion and elimination are essential for your performance.

Beyond these obvious immediate side effects of over-eating, there are health dangers in eating excessive amounts of protein. Excess amino acids cannot be stored as protein, so they are stored as fat and their breakdown and elimination generates a toxic byproduct called urea. Eliminating urea increases water loss and excretion of calcium in urine, which in turn may cause kidney stones and bone loss. Coming from the fitness industry, I am appalled to see the size of protein shakes and the proportions of protein contained in them, which far exceeds the 30g that the body can absorb in one sitting. Remember that almost all food contains some sort of protein so it is unlikely you'd be lacking. Usually, it is the complete opposite. And long-term excess protein intake can lead to kidney and liver damage and weight gain.

Here is how to estimate your minimum daily protein requirement (in grams). Multiply your ideal body weight in lbs by 0.37, or your weight in kilograms by 0.8. This is the number of grams of protein you require each day. Your protein need is: _____.

I weigh 128 lbs, with a daily protein intake of 47g, and I found this worked wonders for me, even working out a solid 15 hours a week as a fitness instructor. *An important point to stress is that eating more protein does not make you build more muscle. (Lifting more does.) Eating excess protein makes you fatter.* Professional body builders (real ones, not people who just lift weights) have slightly higher protein needs but it is a very slight increase: They need 1.0 to 1.2g of protein per kg of body weight compared to 0.8g of protein per kg for normal people. The multiplier would be 0.6 to figure out the number of protein in lbs. If I were a competing body builder, my protein intake would increase from 47g to 77g (128 lbs x 0.6). Far below what people generally believe is needed.

To avoid excess eating, I recommend my clients follow the old Ayurveda advice of eating until they feel satisfied, which means 75% full.

Prescription 4: Reduce your consumption of cooked foods, which are addictive, in favor of raw foods.

Have you ever noticed how hard it is to stop eating cooked foods? Resisting a second or third slice of pizza for instance… Stopping after one little chicken thigh and not have the whole wing… How about eating a pasta dish? Could you quit after an antipasti portion? What happens after that one burger at a BBQ party with friends? Do you go for seconds?

On the other hand, you cannot very easily overdo raw food. How many broccoli, carrots, sprouts, beans, pumpkin seeds, or mangoes can you eat in one sitting really? First, this is because raw foods have a very high nutrient density, which fulfills your body's nutritional needs and turns off the hunger hormone ghrelin. Second, the volume occupied in your stomach by raw foods makes you feel full quickly. And third, the water contained in raw food prevents us eating a large amount (water is the first thing that evaporates in cooking foods) as does the amount of fiber.

Cooked food on the other hand contains far fewer nutrients. As Dr. Gillian McKeith wrote in her book *You Are What You Eat:* "When food is cooked above 118 degrees F, the enzymes are destroyed in full. Most protein is destroyed or converted to forms that are not easily digested when cooked. Cooked food destroys a large majority of the vitamins. It is estimated that 50% of B vitamins (including B12), 97% folic acid and up to 80% of vitamin C is lost. When food is cooked we are often getting 15% of the nutritive value of the food."

This is why, in my opinion, we over-eat cooked foods. The body is starving for nutrition and asking for more and more food until it makes up for its 100% nutrient RDA. So whenever you want to eat cooked food, work with the concepts of warming up your food rather than cooking at high heat for long periods of time. For instance, for stir fry or soups, I always add fresh raw vegetables at the end of the cooking time, just before serving the dish so the veggies preserve their nutrient density.

In addition, there are a number of addictive substances in certain foods. One of my nutrition heroines, Victoria Boutenko, author of numerous books including *12 Steps to Raw Foods,* saved her entire family struck with various ailments by turning everyone onto the raw food diet overnight. In her book, Victoria lists the addictive substances of several foods. She explains:

- "Sugar and foods that contain sugar release endogenous opiates (natural morphine-like chemicals) that induce a sense of pleasure and well-being in the brain". The same opiate chemicals can be found in white bread, cereal, pasta, and other foods made from white flour.

- Meat, poultry and fish contain opioid peptides. In addition, grilled meat contains two further toxic substances (AC and MeAC), which are addictive and found in cigarette smoke. Now hear this! Victoria says: "1g of grilled beef contains 650.8ng of AC and 63.5ng of MeAC, which is the equivalent of eight cigarettes. Now, a small 100g serving of barbecued meat is equal to *800 cigarettes!*" No wonder grilled meat is so popular in the US and consumed daily!

- Milk also contains opioid peptides and is very addictive. (Rightfully so, to keep mother and baby close.) Concentrated milk products like cheese are even more addictive because they contain another addictive substance: salt.

- Salt cravings are really cravings for minerals which are not met. Hence the over-indulgence in the wrong kinds of salt, or a need to balance exposure to excess yin foods (alcohol and sugar topping the list). Sodium is necessary for normal functioning of the human body and people deficient in sodium are not eating enough of the foods that are richest in sodium: dark leafy greens and sea vegetables. That means everyone on the Standard American Diet (SAD). If you eat plants that are rich in sodium salts because they are grown in a nutrient-rich soil, you do not need to salt your food. I challenge you to eliminate salt for a few weeks and discover the natural flavors of your foods with renewed interest.

If you are trying to reduce your intake of the 11 inflammatory foods, you are better to go at it cold turkey, because cooked and processed foods are addictive. Just having a little bit is more torturous!

1.3
COOK AS IF YOUR LIFE DEPENDS ON IT, BECAUSE
IT DOES: THE 10-MINUTE MEAL FOR THE BUSY
PROFESSIONAL.

Learning how to cook and cooking 90% of your meals is
the secret to vibrant health. Unless you carefully control the
cooking process yourself, the food you are eating while you're
out may be over-cooked, old, made with poor quality food,
rancid oils and so on. Of course, there is also the hygiene
issue.

Cooking at home feels rebellious in today's society when de-
livery meals are ordered from our smartphones, but if you
are serious about reaching your goals, your kitchen or hotel
room is the place where you need to concoct your elixirs. As
Aristotle said: "Let Food Be Thy Medicine".

When I traveled around India to learn different Indian cooking traditions, the family I stayed with in Bhubaneshwar
told me about the 'restaurant menu'. When Indians go out
to restaurants with the family, they do not want to eat the
same food they prepare at home (and God knows how delicious homemade Indian food is). So basically, the restaurant
menu includes all these rich, creamy gravy dishes that are not
the daily fare in an Indian home. Rather, they are the 'party'
fares. Think of this next time you order food out or dine in
a restaurant. The restaurant menu is always a 'party menu'.
Real homemade food is much simpler than that and takes 20
minutes to eat, not the 90 minutes that a business lunch or
dinner takes.

If your life is on the road Monday through Thursday, you may
end up eating 'party' meals three times a day for four days, for
a year, or even for a decade unless you take action. The food

at work, airports, hotels, and on airplanes is of poor quality. It is too rich. There are too few fresh organic vegetables, leafy greens and fresh fruits available and, in some circumstances, the food may not even be safe for consumption.

Similarly, working in an office is like having a party meal every day. It's always someone's birthday so there is cake. Then there are always a few catered meals, which include the processed sandwiches, the nutrition-less iceberg salad and the platter of cookies.

Not to mention the assortment of sodas. And finally, the lunch out with co-workers or clients.

You can prepare a delicious meal at home in 10 minutes. Becoming a 10-minute cook is a life-saving skill and it's something I help my readers with by designing and posting sample meal plans on my blog at blog.zenberrymix.com and I include a sample meal plan in appendix 3. Further, the benefits of cooking at home go well beyond the food, as we'll soon discover.

So what are you willing to do to change the situation? Where will you draw the line? How will you recreate the simplicity of a homemade meal where careful attention is given to each ingredient, the cooking method and amount of time you have in a relaxing environment?

1.4
EAT HEALTHILY ON THE ROAD.

When you live on the road, be it one trip per month or weekly journeys, the process to eat healthy remains the same as at home: planning and executing the plan.

Planning before you leave on your trip:

- Make yourself a high-level meal plan (example in appendix 4).

- Surf the internet for restaurants, juice or smoothie bars, for vegan or vegetarian choices and for fulfillment of your menu items.

- Review the restaurant menus in advance and call to ask questions.

- Look for whole foods and farmers market for fresh on-the-go produce.

    › Check wholefoodsmarket.com

    › Try organicconsumers.org/purelink.html for a list of co-ops and natural health food stores.

- At the grocery store, shop for snacks and breakfast items that you can eat in your room, if you cannot resist the hotel breakfast buffet. See a list of snacks, on-the-go grocery items and the recipe of my favorite homemade superfood trail mix in appendices 1 and 2. The trail mix balances bitter and sweet superfoods with the fatty nuts, seeds and exotic coconut. I love the worldly feeling of the trail mix too, which combines ingredients from Asia, US and South America.

- If attending a business dinner function, call the restaurant ahead of time and let them know about your dietary restrictions. Try to eat a healthy snack, resembling a mini meal, before the dinner function so as not to arrive hungry and devour the bread basket, peanuts, chips or pretzels. You will also feel less affected by alcohol and make better choices ordering from the restaurant menu. And remember the point of a business dinner is to socialize and build meaningful relationships. Focus on people rather than the food at the function. You'll make a lasting impression.

• Drink two glasses of water for every one glass of alcohol consumed or skip the liquor entirely for Perrier lemon, Perrier orange or Perrier with fresh berries instead.

EMMA'S STORY

On our way to the hotel, my team and I would take a cab from the airport to the local whole foods store or food coop to stock up on items that we could keep in our rooms or the minibar (which we had asked the hotel to empty beforehand). At other times, we would leave the hotel at 7.00am, drive to the health food store and buy a breakfast that we'd eat there, as well as a lunch salad, a green smoothie and some fresh fruit to snack on. We even had a team coop tote bag that we took proudly to our client site. We would store our food in the fridge, or bring it around with us as we drove from client site to client site in our rental car. To this day, my team has continued this daily practice. It was a win-win situation for us (healthy) and the client (cheap).

Here are a few more of my favorite internet resources to find a healthy restaurant on the road:

- Try eatwellguide.org/localguide for an online directory for family farms, restaurants, markets and more.

- Check happycow.net for a list of health food stores and healthy restaurants.

- You can also use my Dining-Out Questionnaire in appendix 6 to help you order healthy foods at restaurants.

There are a couple of utensils I traveled with to get better control of my health, especially when I got sick or when I wanted to have a 'clean' week:

- A small blender like the NutriBullet went just fine through the TSA security checkpoint in my backpack. I used the NutriBullet to prepare two green smoothies in the morning. One for breakfast and one for later in the day that I would pack in my computer bag. I also used my blender to make an oatmeal drink for breakfast, and sometimes for dinner, when I skipped the team dinner. (Check out some of my breakfast recipes in appendix 5).

- A shaker bottle was useful as a refillable water bottle or a shaker bottle to make and carry liquid shakes around.

- A small Black & Decker rice cooker for one person. Don't laugh! I carried it around throughout the winter to make my own oatmeal breakfast and kichadi dinner in the hotel room. As a nutritionist, I also did three detoxes a year, which required super-simple food intake. I was able to make those meals in my rice cooker and carry it to work in a Kleen Kanteen insulated bottle. I came across two Delta flight attendants making their own foods at the back of the airplane with the same small rice cooker too!

It's worth going the extra mile in planning to see results. Remember your goals! I feel younger and am fitter now than I have ever been in my youth. I am stronger than I was in my athletic college years and haven't been sick in years, not since I implemented this regimen. I'm not even vaccinated against the flu. I used to get four colds a year, the flu and a gastroenteritis every winter when working in Corporate America, even though I was being vaccinated every winter to prevent the flu. Long gone the pain!

As one of my successful clients, Jeff, put it: "You've got to be a badass and stop worrying about what other people think to do what's right for you".

Evidence that your dietary changes are heading in the right direction are: accrued energy in the morning and throughout the day, fewer body aches, more restful sleep, improved digestion, clearer skin and better mental clarity. But depending on where you started from, you may feel worse before you start feeling better.

When your diet improves, the first thing your body does is start to repair and detoxify. You are finally getting out of your way and giving your body a chance to renew itself. As a result, you may experience detoxification symptoms during the first few days or week. The symptoms may be uncomfortable, but they are a normal part of detoxification and they typically subside within a few days. Refrain from taking painkillers, which are toxic to your liver. If you experience any severe symptoms, consult your physician immediately.

Healing reactions in your body associated with eating more of the 11 healthy foods and banning the 11 inflammatory foods may include:

- Headaches

- Mood swings

- Skin rashes (temporary) from your 'derma' flushing toxins

- Gas, diarrhea or constipation from elimination

- Fatigue (so get plenty of sleep!)

- Cravings for the foods you let go

- Toxic hunger such as dizziness, light headedness, stomach cramps and so on (although *real* hunger is not painful and is felt in the mouth and neck)

Please don't give up! These symptoms typically won't last more than a few days, maybe a week. I like to think of the body's detoxification process as a rite of passage towards a better self and the formation of new healthy eating habits. The journey is difficult but oh-so rewarding.

The three foods I know I could be eating for energy (but am not) are:

_____

_____

_____

The foods I depend on from the list of 11 inflammatory foods are:

_____

_____

_____

_____

_____

One food I will start eating over the next two weeks:

_____

One food I will stop eating over the next two weeks:

_____

One new habit I will start in the next two weeks in order to position myself for success:

_____

_____

One old hurtful habit I will stop doing in order to position myself for success:

_____

_____

This will make me stick to my plan and consistently choose the good foods over the bad foods:

_____

_____

_____

Beyond the food... What do I really crave? What's missing most from my life? What is essential to my happiness?

_____

_____

_____

_____

_____

_____

_____

_____

_____

_____

_____

_____

_____

_____

_____

_____

_____

_____

_____

_____

_____

_____

_____

6
MILESTONE 2:
SLEEP FOR CLARITY AND
YOUTHFULNESS

Achieve restful and uninterrupted sleep consistently, night
after night, feeling refreshed and energetic in the morning,
with mental clarity, and emotional calm and stability. Feel
young, light, and spring from your youthful life force.

Are you tired of being tired? If you are a busy and dedicated
worker bee, I suspect you may be chronically exhausted, that
you may wake up in the morning dragging your feet, with a
mental fog, possibly with aches and pain, and dedicating the
first moments of your day trying to shake off the night and
reclaim your focus.

No matter how long you sleep, you feel little energy in the morning and always a little older. Sounds familiar?

Guess what! This is not normal! No matter how hard you work, no matter how old you are, every day when you wake up, you're starting with a clean slate. You're starting afresh.

So how come you're not feeling fresh? How can you enhance the quality of your sleep to make it deeply restorative? What does it feel like to wake up filled with energy, anticipation and excitement for the day?

When was the last time I felt really good waking up in the morning and why was that?

_____
_____
_____
_____
_____
_____
_____
_____

Just like our food is bio-individual, the circumstances that promote restful sleep are unique for each one of us as well, which is why I'll check-in with you and ask a few more questions to help you think through your needs and determine the changes that you need to make around sleep.

The many ways your sleep affects your physical, mental and emotional health... Chronic sleep issues lead to short-term and long-term health issues. In the short term, you crave sugar, caffeine, chemical stimulants to wake up and stay awake longer, taxing your system further, digging a deeper hole and sending you into overdrive. When tired, we eat 25% more food. A sleep-deprived person is on average 30 lbs heavier than a person who routinely sleeps eight hours a night. A study by Eastern Virginia Medical School reported that people who consistently get eight hours of sleep had a body mass index (BMI) 5.5 points lower on average (about 30 lbs difference). This is because, when sleep-deprived, the hunger hormone ghrelin is turned up to overdrive and the satiety hormone leptin is turned off.

Over the medium to long term, you begin to develop mental, emotional and physical health issues. I know you know that, but if you're reading this, you may be stuck and unsure of how to enhance your sleep or make more time for it. So let me further explain what sleep does and how making bedtime a priority, and reorganizing your life around it, will enable you to advance your professional and personal agenda faster, as opposed to reorganizing your sleep around your life.

How sleep works. There basically are two categories of sleep, the quiet sleep and the REM (rapid eye movement) sleep. You alternate between them over the course of 90 minutes. The quiet sleep is made of four gradually deeper stages of sleep and the deepest stage produces physiological changes that boost your immune system. The REM sleep is when you dream. A *Harvard Health Publication* from July 2009 states: "Studies report that REM sleep enhances learning and memory, and contributes to emotional health."

The publication further elaborates: "Sleep disruption, which affects the levels of neurotransmitters and stress hormones, wreaks havoc the brain, impairing thinking and emotional regulation. Insomnia may amplify the effects of psychiatric disorders and vice versa."

In short, lack of sleep makes you asocial, emotionally distant, forgetful, and depresses your immune system. It creates aches in the neck, back and other places in your body.

Research shows a correlation between anxiety disorders, ADHD, depression and other mental health issues and lack of sleep. In fact, one of the first signs of Alzheimer's disease is sleep disruption. Lack of sleep also interferes with your ability to secrete and regulate hormones, specifically DHEA, testosterone and growth hormone, and increases the levels of stress hormone cortisol, which starts a ripple effect of health issues in your body.

Long-term-elevated cortisol levels can be highly dangerous. Research shows that it raises insulin and blood sugar levels, increases visceral fat in the stomach area, lowers thyroid function slowing down the metabolism, blocks testosterone uptake (a week of short sleep can drop testosterone levels by 10-15%), lowers immune function, increases blood pressure, weakens muscle tissue, decreases bone mass and slows down thinking. Are you speechless? Lack of sleep promotes an inflammation-prone environment, related to inflammatory ailments. If you are all revved up in the evening, chances are your cortisol levels are higher than they should be.

The natural daily rhythm of cortisol is high in the morning, gradually lowers as the day goes by, and should be at its lowest in the evening, enabling melatonin to kick in as the sun goes down.

If aging and youthfulness matters to you, you'll be interested to know that your body creates human growth hormone during your sleep, 80% of which is created earlier in the night between 11.00pm and 1.00am. Going to bed early (around

10.00pm) is so essential that the hours of sleep before midnight count double in Traditional Chinese Medicine. It is also in the early hours of the night that your adrenal glands (which secrete cortisol) repair. At night, your body detoxifies and weight loss accelerates. In fact, the better you sleep, the easier it is to lose weight and maintain weight loss. The more sleep-deprived a person is, the higher the inflammation and the fatter you become.

Thinking about my health, I can now see that the following mental, emotional and physical issues I've been experiencing may be linked to an inadequate amount of sleep:

_____

_____

_____

_____

_____

_____

_____

_____

_____

Further, the following bad habits I have likely stem from exhaustion and sleep deprivation:

_____

_____

_____

_____

_____

_____

_____

_____

_____

_____

If I had more energy, giving me back another two hours in the day, I would: *(What have you been missing out on that you'd be able to do? Exercise more? Have more sex? Play longer with your kids after work? Pick up a new hobby?)*

_____

_____

_____

_____

_____

_____

_____

_____

_____

_____

EMMA'S STORY

My breakdown and inability to carry on my professional role and personal life to their fullest potential had everything to do with lack of sleep. It is the lack of sleep that started the snowball effect with food. I let a never-ending list of to-dos and obligations dictate my sleep schedule. Sleep always worked around my travel schedule, nightly client and team dinners, or late nights working at the hotel, yet still getting up early to exercise. The weekends were not restful, but filled with activities to make up for the time away from home, catching up with my partner, our friends and finding time for personal projects, and contributing my time to professional boards, all of which ate up my sleep time.

How I used my time was entirely up to me but, back then, I did not see it that way. I felt I had to do this and that. I had no choice. But of course, I did. Funny how our mind keeps us locked in powerful current habits or identity. Like a status symbol, mine was that of the New York busy bee, gifted with superhuman productivity, able to deliver on everything almost simultaneously and being consumed by perfectionism. No time to rest or sleep with what is expected of me. And yes, I'm very happy!! Why do you ask?

So how do you break the no-sleep spiral and reclaim restful sleep?

Let me start with asking you a few more questions to determine what your ideal sleep pattern would look like:

The number of hours' sleep per night that makes me feel deeply rested is _____.

If I sleep less than _____, I feel edgy and reach for sugar and caffeine the next day.

I feel the first calling for bedtime in the evening (yawning, sleepiness, craving for energy to stay up) at _____.

Therefore, my ideal bedtime is _____.

My natural wake-up time on the days I don't use an alarm clock is _____.

When I feel tired, this is what prevents me from going to bed:

_____

_____

_____

_____

Armed with this knowledge, here are my prescriptions for restful sleep.

1	Reorganize your life around your sleep schedule.
2	Identify and address any sleep disorders that prevent you from sleeping through the night.
3	Take a nap when you are tired.
4	Create your own sleep ritual and implement it consistently.

Prescription 1: Reorganize your life around your sleep schedule.

To reorganize your life to accommodate your ideal bedtime, leverage your new belief system. You designed it to support the goals you're marching towards.

What would it take for you to go to sleep at your ideal bedtime and how will you execute on that plan?

EMMA'S STORY

I discovered that my ideal bedtime was 9.30pm. Work day, weekend, vacation, it does not matter. I feel my best throughout the day when I am in bed at 9.30pm. I also discovered that I need a solid eight hours of sleep, but it comes second after my bed-time. Sleeping from midnight to 8.00am does not make feel as good as sleeping eight hours between 9.30pm and 5.30am, my preferred wake-up time.

In fact, a couple of nights going to bed after 11.00pm

shatters me and begins to trigger my auto-immune markers. It took me over two years to resuscitate my adrenal glands from a deep pit of exhaustion and vanquish insomnia. Going past my bedtime more than two or three nights a week does not sit well with me.

So how did I, a management consultant traveling for work, launching a start-up and going to school full-time, get to bed at 9.30pm and sleep for eight hours of restful sleep?

I reorganized my life around my sleep schedule, which boosted my career and increased the quality of my relationships.

In order to be done in time, I had to become a better consultant and leader quickly. Having less time to dedicate to any given task has an incredible ability to teach you how to concentrate your power on the task at hand. I stopped multi-tasking (which was my old modus operandi).

I went straight to the core of the matter, focusing on the best value to deliver to the client and killing scope creep. Getting straight to the point and delivering the right service the first time because there isn't time for rework requires you to really listen and understand what the client, partner, or team member needs. It also teaches you to work in close collaboration with your team and your client to co-create the best solution. I was asking better questions, collaborating better through the development process, and became excellent at setting boundaries. I became a champion of effective delegation, supporting and holding others accountable for their share of the work. My personal standards de facto skyrocketed as a direct result of my laser focus. Powerful concentration means saying no to what is not directly of concern in the matter at hand, or otherwise put, holding boundaries. If I said yes, my standards would have had to lower, my efficiency would have suffered and ultimately my sleep would again have been last on my list.

So I said no a lot but delivered better and faster. In the end, I contributed more to the company's bottom line, my clients' success, my team's growth and development, and towards myself because I had more time for the things I wanted to do and activities that made me feel good.

One of the first things I cut was my social life on the road. I reduced it to one night a week, even if I had several trips scheduled in one week. I allowed myself to pass my bedtime only once, so I had to make choices. I also empowered the managers and seniors in my team to take turns in creating evening activities without me, not always geared around dinner, or to lead the night out. Soon, a monthly schedule was set. On one particular project, the men took the team out to see the local baseball team play. The following week, the women took the team, guys included, out for a manicure-pedicure. The week after that, an associate invited the team to his home for a delicious gourmet dinner cooked by his mom visiting from India. And so it went on.

The lesson I learned is that, once you begin to focus on yourself, life falls into place the right way. The people around you take on new roles and responsibilities. Everything turns out for the best. It is when you sacrifice yourself, by denying your need for restful sleep, or exercise or cooking time, that you begin to lower yourself to sub-standards of living, which permeate other areas of your life: your quality of work, your career opportunities, and your relationships.

By putting me and my health first, I gave myself the means to reach all of my goals and the speed of growth was spectacular. I did not even need to apologize or justify anything. I just did what I had to do to be in bed at 9.30pm. By taking care of myself, I was de facto giving permission to others to do the same. What a powerful ripple effect of health.

Thinking outside the box, without making excuses, the list of changes I could make to get adequate sleep include:

_____
_____
_____
_____
_____
_____
_____
_____
_____
_____
_____
_____
_____
_____
_____
_____

Prescription 2: Identify and address any sleep disorders that prevent you from sleeping through the night.

Getting to bed is half the battle. The other half is falling and staying asleep. Chronic sleep issues affect about 15% of the US adult population. These can include snoring, sleep apnea, insomnia and restless leg syndrome. Consult a physician to establish a strategy to overcome your sleep issues.

The diet and lifestyle changes proposed in this book will also have a definite effect on any and all of these. Creating a sleep ritual may help you achieve quality sleep faster.

Prescription 3: Take a nap when you are tired.

EMMA'S STORY

> You can sleep-train your body. In high school, I trained my body to nap for 15 minutes anytime, anywhere, to prepare for my last year of study, the gruesome months leading up to the French Baccalauréat, then after that to sustain four years of competitive university studies at the Institut d'Etudes Politiques. This is one of the best things I've ever learned. To this day, I can still fall sleep anytime, anywhere, in a few seconds and wake up by myself 10 to 13 minutes later feeling completely energized, clear-headed, and ready for hours more productivity.
>
> I've napped at work too when working from my employer's office, sneaking into the 'quiet room' (the lactation room for new moms) whenever I found my productivity diminishing, typically around 2.00pm. Napping at work is an acceptable practice in some countries in

Southern Europe and parts of Asia. I remember visiting an office in Taipei, Taiwan, at lunchtime. Suddenly, a bell, which could be heard throughout town, rang. The workers in the open space switched off the lights, each pulled a pillow from under their desks, and proceeded to sleep with their head laying on the pillow on their desk. I retreated to the pantry with my friend Charlotte, the only room with a light on, and we were hushed because our whispers were still too loud for the sleepers… After the lunch hour, the lights were turned back on, pillows hidden and everyone went back to their work on the phones, typing on computers, as if nothing had happened.

Napping dramatically increases learning, memory and awareness. And it feels really good. So how long should you nap for? An article published in *Natural Society* summarizing research on the topic says that a power nap of 10 to 20 minutes is best to refresh your mind, and increase your energy and alertness. It enables you to get right back to work upon waking. Staying asleep longer can lead to grogginess. Whereas 60-minute naps are good for memory boosting. Longer naps, around 90 minutes, are good for those people who just don't get enough sleep at night. It's a complete sleep cycle and can improve emotional and procedural memory (riding a bike, learning the piano) and creativity. I've seen it work well for people who work night shifts or double shifts. Napping is also fantastic after a hard physical effort to recover physically.

I find that in a busy life, where no two days look alike, napping is an excellent complement to a good night's sleep.

Prescription 4: Create your own sleep ritual and implement it consistently.

A sleep ritual is another tool that can help you fall asleep faster and stay asleep throughout the night, especially when traveling and sleeping in unfamiliar environments.

A sleep ritual is highly personal and so your ritual will differ from my ritual. To help you create one, chose practices that you find relaxing mentally, emotionally and physically.

These are some factors to consider:

- *Establish good sleep hygiene.* Good sleep hygiene is the sum of tips and practices surrounding bedtime. The ones I find most effective are: keeping the bedroom pitch black, reserving the bedroom for sleep and sex exclusively, which means removing TV, electronics, work and even food from the bedroom, going to bed and waking up at the same time (plus or minus one hour) every day of the week, keeping the temperature cool, no higher than 70 degrees F, keeping the bedroom clean and orderly, and disconnecting from all electronics 30 to 60 minutes before bedtime.

- *Establish good dietary habits.* The 11 bad foods discussed in the previous chapter have been shown to undermine the quality of sleep. Which ones affect you the most depends on your bio-individuality, of which you have gained awareness by now.

A special note on alcohol... While it depresses the nervous system and makes you feel tired helping you to fall asleep, when the effects wear off, you will wake up. Is that true in your case? If so, that's one more reason to reserve the bottle for special occasions. The time and amount that you eat will also affect the quality of your sleep. I recommend to my clients to stop eating three hours before bedtime in order to go to sleep on an empty stomach. It reduces indigestion, and frees energy for the body to tackle other repair, rebuild and detox tasks overnight. Further, it enhances the quality of sleep (less bloating, acid reflux, gas, waking up in the middle of the night and pain in the belly). Dinner should be light, more like a supper (supplement), to hold you overnight without overburdening you.

- *Relaxation techniques.* Incorporate one or two practices that help you slow down and relax your mind and your body. Examples include: meditation, deep breathing exercises, gentle stretching, progressive muscle relaxation (alternately tensing and releasing muscles). Relaxation techniques help counter anxiety and racing thoughts. They slow down the heart rate and lower the body temperature, connecting the mind with the body, releasing tension and possibly pain in the body. This is the subject of a bigger conversation about slowing down that we'll tackle in Milestone 5.

- *Emotional support.* Much of the time, what keeps us up at night are our thoughts and emotions like anxiety, fear, guilt, remorse, regrets, and grief. Establishing a ritual and a support structure that enables you to acknowledge, release or even simply share your emotions with someone can make all the difference for the quality of your sleep. (We'll tackle this in Milestone 4). For people unable to fall asleep because they are preoccupied by more serious depression, anxiety, and other dysfunctional behaviors, cognitive behavioral therapy is a psychotherapeutic approach that can help build more confidence and create better sleep.

- *Exercise daily.* Daily exercise helps people fall asleep faster, spend more time in deep sleep, and awaken less often during the night. More on the topic of exercise in Milestone 3.

Take a minute now to think about what you are doing right when it comes to going to bed, as well as how you'd like to change your habits.

Here are the habits I currently have which do not support me to go to sleep at my ideal bedtime, or support restful uninterrupted sleep:

_____

_____

_____

_____

_____

_____

_____

Here is what my new sleep ritual looks like:

_____

_____

_____

_____

_____

_____

_____

_____

_____

In conclusion, sleep is the next domino in the GDN blueprint after your food. Without adequate sleep, you won't feel your best and may be drawn into sabotaging your diet for a quick energy fix. Profound chemical imbalances in your body will deteriorate your physical, mental and emotional health. In my experience, all the components of goal-directed nutrition (diet, exercise, supportive relationships and slowing down) are founded on a long night of uninterrupted sleep.

7
MILESTONE 3:
EXERCISE FOR STRENGTH AND LONGEVITY

Exercise to increase focus on goals, for energy, for better sleep and vibrant health; to feel strong and confident; to increase self-esteem, to rejuvenate, prevent illness and live longer; to manage travel stress and avoid jetlag.

You know exercise is good for you, but you don't have time to get to the gym or go for a run. Am I right? Maybe your body is out of shape, aching, or you're recovering from an injury, so afraid to start exercising again. I get it. Would you like to find a way to get back into it? Read on.

EMMA'S STORY

Exercise has always played a big role in my life. It started with my love of horses, touring France during school breaks to watch dressage performances with my mother, a talented equestrian who imparted her passion on me. After years of riding and preparing to certify as an equestrian instructor, I suffered a severe back injury, never to ride again.

So I turned to my second love, the ocean. I started instructing for the French Federation of Sailing at 19 on the Atlantic Sea. I continued through college, where I took up a four-year elective course in body-building and fitness. Today, I hold a personal trainer certification from the US National Academy of Sports Medicine and several other diplomas and have been teaching about 15 fitness classes a week since 2004.

I built my own personal training studio, a long-time dream of mine, and co-created a competitive cycling team promoting healthy eating and clean performance. My favorite classes to teach are aqua-cycling, indoor cycling, TRX, Jillian Michaels BODYSHRED™, Indoboard, BOSU® Bootcamp, heavy weight training, Kangoo Jumps and my 30-minute core class. I love riding my bikes out in nature, and walking on the beach. One of my favorite activities, when I used to live in Manhattan, was walking the 40 minutes to work every morning from the Upper West Side, diagonally across Central Park and down Fifth Avenue to 42nd street where PwC is headquartered.

> My favorite exercise DVD is the Blissology Project, a yoga and meditation practice for every day of the week, staged in beautiful Bali and a great way to workout in a hotel room. As a corporate employee and now as an entrepreneur, I work out in the morning and at night, and do a few additional walks or bursts of activity during the day. In my opinion, the key to sticking with exercise is flexibility, variety, moderation and self-awareness.

In goal-directed nutrition, exercise is connected to strength and longevity and an essential key element to feeding your success. Let me show you how to create an active lifestyle that feels good.

Here is a summary of the exercise prescriptions covered in this chapter.

1	Be clear on your goals, and how exercise can help you reach them, if at all.
2	Don't overestimate how much exercise you need, as a little bit goes a long way.
3	Adopt a form of exercise that is right for your body type.
4	Be realistic and practical when starting your exercise program.
5	Adopt an integrative training approach to balance your needs and keep it fresh.
6	Plan exercise in your schedule and hold yourself accountable.

Prescription 1: Be clear on your goals, and how exercise can help you reach them, if at all.

The majority of the people I come across are exercising to lose weight or to prepare for an athletic event. My classes are jam-packed in January coinciding with new year's resolutions around weight loss and in May and June to get beach-ready. These people soon lose motivation and stop coming. I would too if weight loss was the main (or only) reason for exercising.

Research has long proven that you cannot exercise your way out of a bad diet and that weight loss is not a function of balancing calories in and calories out, but eating the right foods, getting adequate sleep and keeping stress and inflammation down.

Therefore, the key to motivating you to start exercising again and stick with it is to select viable goals that exercise can help you achieve, with tangible measurable results. Personally, I would not be where I am today, successful in business, in love, and vibrantly healthy and happy without exercise. This is why I exercise:

- It gives me physical pleasure. I feel good and happy when I sweat.

- It makes me feel stronger and more confident. After an exercise session, I feel empowered to brave my fears and take risks to further my goals. I make decisions faster with more assurance.

- I feel more creative after an exercise session. My brain neurons have been shaken up and I see things from a different vantage point.

- It makes me feel and look younger. Exercise is the ultimate fountain of youth. Studies lasting many years have consistently shown that being active cuts the risk of premature death by about 50% for men and women alike.

- It gives me tons of energy, which I need to go forth with my career plans and life aspirations. I feel more adventurous after a particularly brainy workout, which required the use of multiple skills: cardio, agility, speed, balance, strength, flexibility, etc.

- It keeps me disease- and infection-free, as moderate workouts temporarily rev-up the immune system by increasing the aggressiveness or capacity of immune cells. I have not had the flu or a cold in years despite living in a dirty crowded city where everyone else gets sick and being exposed to more germs when traveling.

- It helps me sleep because it keeps my stress under control and releases tension in my body. Regular aerobic exercise lowers levels of stress hormones.

- It curbs my food cravings. Exercise helps maintain healthy blood-sugar levels by increasing the cells' sensitivity to insulin and by controlling weight. If I start thinking about food, it's a sign that I need to get up and move to energize.

- It keeps my body pain- and ache-free despite several serious back injuries and advanced arthritis in my back. It keeps my soft tissues 'juicy', warm, and flexible through their complete range of motion. It's only when I move less or skip exercise for as little as two days that my aches and pains come back, probably from growing stiff and tense from lack of movement.

- It maintains my general health impeccably. Perfect blood tests. Exercise also raises 'good' HDL cholesterol and lowers blood pressure, and lessens the risk of heart attacks by reducing arterial inflammation. My resting heart rate dropped from 120 bpm at the height of Graves' disease, down to my old normal 60 bpm, and down again to 40 bpm today. My breathing capacity is much greater and my VO2 max has greatly improved, as has my tolerance for high-intensity training.

- Exercise also helps relieve jetlag and stay awake in the new time zone. I highly recommend you hit the gym or go for a walk when you arrive at your destination. Exercise raises cortisol levels, which helps you wake up.

All of these goals are instantly measurable in terms of: energy, pain management, controlled appetite, mental clarity, levels of self-esteem, blood tests, resting heart rate, VO2 max, endurance levels, speed, agility, and range of motion in your limbs.

Exercise is the best tool for becoming stronger and maintaining your youth, both mentally and physically. Understanding the aging process better may further motivate you to exercise a lot more than you have, or differently than you have.

Your body's proper posture and youthful appearance depend on your muscles' ability to hold your bones, joints in alignment. Nothing screams more of old age than a hunched-over posture, stiffness, and lack of range of motion in your limbs, regardless of how old you really are. We've all seen people in their 40s who moved and looked like a 20-year-old. (I live with one. It's so much fun!) Likewise, we've seen people in their 20s who appeared 20 years older.

As we age, most people begin to lose *muscle mass* after the age of 30 and *bone density* after the age of 40. Bone density peaks between the ages of 25 and 35. Eventually as we age our bones shrink and become less dense. Even new bones grow thinner. Unfortunately, you cannot back pedal in time. Rather, you need to find a way to maintain what you do have now. And the sooner the better.

When you lose your muscle mass or when unnatural posture caused by, say, improper sitting occurs, you can no longer hold yourself well and eventually develop neck, back, shoulder and leg pain. The effects of losing muscle mass include a decrease in strength, greater susceptibility to injury, and an increase in body fat. This physical deterioration has repercussions in your mental and emotional being. You begin losing self-confidence and hiding a body you find less attractive, robbing the world of your talents.

What's even worse, thinking about the state of our youth today, is that sedentary individuals can begin to lose muscle mass *as early as their mid-twenties.* Human beings can lose up to 2% of muscle mass per year, eventually losing as much as 50% of muscle mass in the course of a lifetime. Based on my experience, building more muscle mass after age 30 is very difficult and requires more effort than for someone in their 20s.

By starting earlier rather than later, you will increase your likelihood of *maintaining* greater muscle mass as you age.

When done properly, exercise improves strength levels, develops bone density, increases metabolism, decreases injury, and improves body image.

I am also convinced that the better you are at exercise, the better you'll be at everything else in life. If you're already hugely successful in life but lacking in the exercise department, give it a serious try. You have no idea how much more amazing your current life can be! Now it's your turn. Why do you want or need to exercise?

The reasons I want to exercise are: *(list a minimum of five reasons)*

_____

_____

_____

_____

_____

_____

_____

_____

_____

_____

_____

_____

_____

_____

_____

_____

_____

_____

Prescription 2: Don't overestimate the amount of exercise you need, as a little bit goes a long way.

There's plenty of research evidencing that short but frequent bouts of exercise can yield plenty of health benefits. Consider the following findings:

- A study published by the *American Journal of Sports Medicine* in 2006 showed that short walks after dinner were more effective than long exercise sessions in reducing the amount of fat and triglyceride levels in the bloodstream after a hearty meal.

- Research published in the *Journal of Epidemiology and Community Health* showed that short bouts of exercise helped lower blood pressure as well as shave inches off the hips and waistline.

- In a study published in *Preventive Medicine* in 2006, researchers found that multiple workout sessions as short as 6 minutes apiece could help sedentary adults reach fitness goals similar to those achieved by working out for 30 minutes at a time.

- A study published in the *American Journal of Health Promotion* in 2012 found that, for preventing weight gain, the intensity of the activity matters more than its duration. Accumulated higher-intensity physical activity bouts of under 10 minutes proved highly beneficial, supporting the notion that 'every minute counts'.

As such, whether you exercise 30 minutes a day (minimum recommended amount by the US Government) in one exercise session or three times 10 minutes, both are equally beneficial. I'll be honest with you, because we are talking about taking your life to the next level, I recommend you gradually increase your amount of exercise to three or four short intense bouts of exercise a day as well as longer periods of exercise a few times a week.

Working out for 60 to 90 minutes and working out for 10 minutes develop different aptitudes, both of which are desired to build the well-rounded business professional that you wish to be. You want to react and decide quickly, withstand high levels of stress with less damage. (Whether caused by physical or mental stress, the effects on your nervous system are similar, so intense exercise can be great training). But you also want to last the distance, to be able to pace yourself to witness the seeds blossom that you planted and nurtured. Endurance work teaches you how to pace yourself.

In addition, as a side note, your body uses different fuels for different exercise intensity: a greater percentage of fatty acids at lower heart rate and higher percentage of sugar at higher intensity levels (and then chemicals at the highest anaerobic levels). This is a simplification of a complex process but this means that you want to make sure you don't become a sugar junkie by continuously working out at max intensity. Most of the recreational exercisers who take my classes work out too hard, too many times a week without periodizing their training and feast on sugary drinks and gels to power their workout, and overeat because they feel overly hungry with huge swings of blood sugar. Doing so compromise their gut health and digestion. (More on this coming up). Working out too much leads to injuries, increased stress-related inflammation, weight gain, and fitness plateau.

Prescription 3: Adopt a form of exercise that is right for your body type.

There are infinite ways to exercise and the way you choose to exercise is bio-individual. There is not one size of exercise that fits all. Indeed, in the tradition of Ayurveda, each dosha (body type) is prescribed a different modality of exercise to balance out their physical, emotional, mental, and behavioral nature:

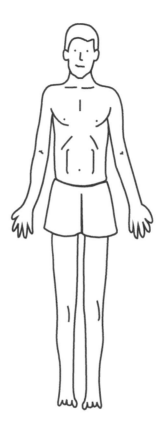

The thin and bony people, tall or short, are the Vata or winter body types. They traditionally have low body fat, delicate bones, a hard time gaining weight, and a volatile and overactive mind. They are attracted to physically vigorous forms of exercise but should rather focus on weight-lifting and rock-climbing to increase bone density, and gentle forms of exercise like yoga, Pilates, swimming, tai chi and walking to ground and appease their minds.

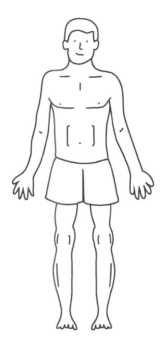

The people with medium build, and developed and proportionate musculature are the Pitta or summer body types. They traditionally overheat, are prone to inflammation, sweat a lot, have a strong metabolism, easily gain and lose weight and are aggressive. They are attracted to action sports and competitive activities. Yet, what they need the most to balance their nature is calming exercise like swimming, cycling, walking, tai chi, Pilates and the less heating, vigorous forms of yoga like hatha yoga.

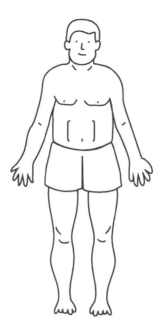

People with the larger body type, heavy bones, broad frame, strong and proportionate are the Kapha or spring body types. They have a tendency to gain weight and hold on to fat and water. They are cool, graceful, slow, and at times lethargic. They are great powerful athletes when in shape, but avoid physical exertion. They need a serious kick in the butt to get going and need to engage in vigorous cardiovascular exercise like running, spinning, hiking and the more vigorous forms of yoga like hot yoga, Bikram or vinyasa flow.

Prescription 4: Be realistic and practical when starting your exercise program.

Exercising is a lifestyle. Just like brushing your teeth, it needs to become a daily routine if you are committed to feeding your success and making it big. Like any lifestyle changes, it takes some time to form a new habit, about six months. So be realistic, and set your expectations for the long haul.

Begin with focusing on carving out time daily, for 15 minutes of movement. Don't worry much about what to do as much as focusing on time management. You could be walking around the block, going up and down the stairs of your building, or dancing to your three favorite songs.

It does not have to be perfect, but it must be safe, fun and a daily commitment. Remember your goals. Everything you do every day has the potential to take you closer to your goal. Exercise is one of those things. It is when you become rigid about exercise and mentally fixated on one format (the gym) that it becomes difficult to honor your commitment.

Prescription 5: Adopt an integrative training approach to balance your needs and keep it fresh.

The National Academy of Sports Medicine defines Integrated Training as: "A concept that incorporates all forms of training in an integrated fashion as part of a progressive system." In essence, one should design and execute a training routine that includes different exercise modalities such as flexibility training, cardiorespiratory training, core strengthening, balance training, resistance training, reactive training and, for people partaking in team sports, speed, agility and quickness training.

When practicing all these different exercise modalities over the course of a week or two in a progressive fashion (increasingly more challenging), your body and your mind build new neurological connections making you stronger, sharper, more confident and radiant in every aspect of your life.

I have worked with many clients who had lost their motivation and inspiration for life, were less and less active, feeling more and more aches and pains. As their bodies deteriorated, they became narrow-minded, did not have any desires, dreams or goals. They were basically following the motions of life, growing increasingly bored and depressed. Within five sessions of an integrative training program, they were regaining their excitement for life, cheered up, their vision expanded, their aches and pains gone, and generally felt more social and joyful. Of course, physical strength, stamina, balance, agility and flexibility improved as well, making them fitter for life.

Another benefit of following an integrative training protocol is variety. People doing the same exercise routine over and over again eventually get bored or burned out. When an exercise routine is repetitive, too intense or imbalanced, it leads to injuries, pain and eventually people stop exercising. Then every time they try again, they hurt themselves again. But when following an integrative approach as part of a progressive system, exercise is periodized around the year (divided into small progressive steps), following different intensity modalities, to prevent injury and maximize results.

When you look at exercise as a way to shape your physical and mental strength, and bring about emotional stability, you understand why spending a little time exercising each day can add up to some major transformation within weeks, then months, and of course some 365 exercise bouts over the course of a year!

Below are the objectives of the main training modalities and examples of exercises for each. Complete the list with your personal resolutions by listing the form of exercise you enjoy doing or may want to explore.

Flexibility Training

Objective: To maintain or reclaim normal length of your body's soft tissues to enable full range of motion around your joints. It includes different stretching exercises targeting all sides of your body (known as planes of motion).

Examples: yoga, barre

Your resolution (what/when):

_____

_____

Cardio Training

Objective: To develop (stress) the cardiorespiratory system by engaging in physical activities that increase the heart rate at different levels (also called heart rate zones).

Examples: walking, jogging, cycling, rowing, swimming, hiking, spinning, dance, high intensity interval training (HIIT)

Your resolution (what/when):

_____

_____

Core Training

Objective: To strengthen the abdominal, back, hip and gluteal muscles (referred to as the lumbo-pelvic-hip complex), which is the center of the body and the starting point for any movement to be safely executed.

Examples: Core training, Pilates

Your resolution (what/when):

_____

_____

Resistance Training

Objective: To increase the body's functional capacity to adapt to stressors, like body weight or a dumbbell.

Examples: Weight-lifting, Plyometrics, TRX suspension training, kettlebells, rock-climbing, bouldering, P90X DVDs

Your resolution (what/when):

_____

_____

Balance Training

Objective: To increase your ability to sustain or maintain your body's stability or center of gravity over its base of support in any circumstance. It includes using training modalities, which challenge your internal stabilization mechanism by getting you off-centered. This is brain training at its best as it stimulates your body's proprioceptors (which situate you in your environment) and mechanoreceptors (responding to mechanical forces, prompting movement). In a nutshell, it teaches your brain to think faster and activate your muscle fibers faster, increasing your reflexes.

Examples: BOSU¬Æ, half foam roll, Airex pad, Dyna Disc, Indoboard, floor with one-legged exercises, yoga

Your resolution (what/when):

_____

_____

Note that you can further push your brain and neuromuscular system with reactive training, speed, agility and quickness training (not covered here as more advanced and not needed for everyone).

Prescription 6: Plan exercise in your schedule and hold yourself accountable.

The first step to holding yourself accountable is to schedule the exercise in your calendar and have a back-up plan if your day does not unfold as expected. Remain flexible and see the big picture: an active lifestyle.

Your calendar should include appointments for formal exercise set-ups, as well as highlight other opportunities throughout the day to be active and schedule those in too:

- Circle client appointments you could walk to and create buffer time in your calendar to allow for that physical activity;

- Take the stairs instead of the elevators at the office;

- Walk the airport terminal;

- Stretch in the airplane every hour (unless you're sleeping);

- Consider small bursts of intensity training in the office, as little as a song lasting 5 to 10 minutes could energize you;

- Have backup plans.

EMMA'S STORY

In my corporate job, when a team member would say, "I'm going to get a coffee. Anyone need anything?" I would say, "Pause. Let's exercise first." The team would get up in the conference room at our client site and begin to follow my four-minute energizer exercise routine. Then everyone would sit down again and get back to work. The coffee trip all forgotten.

At the end of the year, during a three 12-hour day marathon meeting with Human Resources, partners and directors to evaluate the employees for rating and promotion, I would make everyone get up and do cardio kickboxing and a standing stretching session when people started to feel the bagel and cream cheese calling from the corner table.

At a leadership meeting gathering 50 partners and managing directors, I facilitated a workout session and taught them how to massage the tension out of their back, shoulders and glutes using a little ball.

All these bursts of exercise instantly changed the energy in the room. People's moods were uplifted. The temperature rose in their bodies. And of course, people became instantly more social and pleasant with one another!

I wish people felt less self-conscious about starting to exercise in the workplace, not worrying so much about what others might think and lightening up a bit. It is really easy to put together a little routine that can be performed standing and even seated by your desk and executed safely. It could even become a company-wide effort. It would make you feel better for sure and bring a smile to your co-workers' and clients' faces, which is a great thing!

8
MILESTONE 4:
TEAM-UP FOR EMOTIONAL
SUPPORT AND CONNECTION

Build a network of nurturing relationships which supports
the execution of your business and personal goals, prevents
isolation, depression and anxiety, helps you cope with stress,
tough times and worries, and lets you explore your emotions
safely. Learn how to own your emotions for better results
and connection.

Successful people don't get to the top alone, even though
from the outside they look self-made. Successful professionals rely on an army of supportive people to make it to the
top and stay there. The better connected you are, the more

doors will open for you, and the greater your success will be. Conversely, if you are surrounded by negative, envious, incompetent or overly demanding people, the 'energy suckers' as I call them, you're in trouble.

Just as food, sleep and exercise feed us, relationships feed our human hearts and souls. They are an integral part of GDN and your blueprint to feed success. They come in many shapes - friends, family, co-workers - and make life extraordinary. At work, building relationships with different kinds of mentors is crucial. Personally, I had three or four different mentors in Corporate America:

- An informal mentor to learn about the subject matter I was consulting on;

- Another informal mentor for the Pharmaceuticals and Life Sciences industry;

- Another one, called a relationship partner, to connect me with leadership and help me move up the ladder;

- A formal career coach with whom I felt comfortable sharing my career, as well as life challenges, and asking for support any time of the day.

I also built an external professional network to open new doors and opportunities. It helped me develop additional knowledge, create a reputation in the marketplace, gain new clients, identify and recruit new employees, and accelerate my career advancement.

In addition to connection, building nurturing relationships provides you with emotional support. This aspect cannot be underestimated or overlooked. The road to success can feel lonely. Pursuing one's vision may not be understood by others and it takes mental and emotional toughness to stay the course and execute it. As an entrepreneur who created her business, Goji Fitness, from scratch, it all started with my vision and self-powered execution against that vision. I experienced excitement, rejection, doubt, and fear. Having someone to talk to and having nurturing relationships in my life helped me persevere through the rough patches and make it happen.

As a business consultant, traveling for work is isolating. On the road, family and friends are missed. I sometimes felt estranged or disconnected from the people I loved and it cost me several relationships. Understanding emotions and emotional needs, and communicating and fulfilling those needs is essential to feeding success.

Here are two prescriptions to increase emotional support and connection:

1	Assess current relationships and make the necessary changes to surround yourself with nurturing people. Let go of toxic relationships.
2	Explore and tap into your emotions to improve your life and connect more deeply with others.

Prescription 1: Assess your current relationships and make the necessary changes to surround yourself with nurturing people and let go of toxic relationships.

So who's on your team?

The people I enjoy being around and who support me are:

_____

_____

_____

_____

_____

How often do I spend time with them?

_____

_____

_____

_____

_____

The people who are toxic in my life and stress me out are: (Go on... Write it down!)

_____

_____

_____

_____

_____

How often am I in contact with them?

_____

_____

_____

_____

_____

EMMA'S STORY

The first time that I took a hard look at the relationships in my life was in the midst of my meltdown, when I was in need of emotional, mental and physical support. I wish I had spent time earlier cleaning up the relationships in my life because I discovered the hard way, by knocking on doors asking for help, who had my back and who didn't.

The thing with driven busy professionals is that, while we're great at building teamwork and delegating for the most part, we never ask for help with personal matters until it's too late. We push and hustle through.

Thinking back, I realize that I may not have burned out and taken such a big step backwards in my life had I surrounded myself with more of the right people and let go of the wrong people who were wasting my time and energy: I would have chosen to work for different team leaders, different clients; I would have ended the relationship with my then-boyfriend earlier; I would have spent time with good friends and called my parents more often despite the distance, as well as seeking out their advice when my heart felt heavy or when I was worried.

Burning out is a physical meltdown, which usually happens in conjunction with serious mental and emotional stress. The mind and the way we feel has great power over the body.

Mental and emotional stress is very high for people like us who work long hours, in a competitive environment and travel frequently, but we do not easily acknowledge our need to talk about it, nor do we realize there is a need. This puts a strain on our health, and our marital and family relationships, which are already aggravated with travel distance and jetlag. In short, it puts a cap on our happiness.

Who do you speak to when you feel very happy, when you want to celebrate any achievement, big or small?

_____

_____

_____

_____

Who do you speak with when you feel scared, worried, anxious?

_____

_____

_____

_____

What are your emotional needs right now?

_____

_____

_____

_____

To feed success, you must build nurturing and supportive relationships. This means deciding who's on your team and, equally importantly, who should *not be*.

The most supportive people in my life, those I can share shameful and painful experiences with, at any time of the day or night, without fear of judgment, those who I trust to tell me the truth and help me out are:

_____

_____

The toxic relationships in my life that I should distance myself from are:

_____

_____

_____

The immediate next steps I should take to improve the relationships in my life are:

_____

_____

_____

_____

_____

_____

Prescription 2: Explore and tap into your emotions to improve your life and to connect more deeply with others.

Feelings and emotions are manifestations of your instincts, your intuition, telling you whether something is awesome, or whether it's off and you need to make a decision to feel comfortable again. Emotions provide valuable information, like a compass in our life. By increasing your emotional intelligence, you'll be able to take your relationship-building skills to the next level and deeply connect with people who fill you with great happiness.

What opportunities would life hold if I was the master of my emotional experience and had the power to navigate any situation?

_____

_____

_____

_____

_____

This is the burning question my friend, Anne Koller and her company TAPIN Inc. (thetapin.org), has set out to explore and conquer. With her permission, I'd like to share with you a couple of her tools to help you delve into the highs and lows of what it means to be human, emotional beings. In doing so, you'll better understand your own emotional experience, or 'emotion code' as Anne calls it, build genuine connections with others and find real power to harness your natural creative edge and innovative drive.

Through immersive workshops and interactive experiences, TAPIN helps groups and organizations of all sizes and diversities navigate the tidal wave of human emotion that accompanies communication, connection and engagement challenges inherent in doing business. TAPIN exposes, explores, and turns the long-standing 'elephant in the room' into an opportunity to increase your level of awareness, freedom, creativity and happiness.

TAPIN's tailored experiences give you permission to be the detective in your own experience, investigating each emotion like a new data point to better understand your emotion code and remove mental barriers, fears and anxieties to ultimately be a more connected, aware and successful leader.

Let's practice with two exercises that TAPIN designed and shared with me for your benefit:

Exercise 1: Feeling connected and dealing with difficult emotions.

Goals: Create different thought patterns around your emotions.

Instill compassion and trust with your mind and body in order to become more aware and focused on how you feel.

Exercise: Whenever you experience an emotion that is uncomfortable—anger, resentment, guilt, fear, envy—touch your thumb to each finger in turn. Start with your index finger and move to your pinky. As you touch each finger, say one of the below mantras (or another one that resonates with you). Do this as often as needed throughout your day. Continue the practice for 40 days.

- Emotions are my teachers

- I trust my emotions

- I open to emotions

- I am open emotionally

- I am emotionally connected

Exercise 2: A meditation to create awareness, explore and own your emotions.

- *Goals:* The purpose of this exercise, which is executed like a meditation, is to enable you to investigate your emotions like a detective. In doing so, you will better understand them and own your emotional experience, controlling its outcome on your life. If you eat candy every time you feel anxious, acknowledging your anxiety, exploring and understanding it will enable you to consciously address the reasons of your anxiety and keep you off sugar.

- *Pause:* Find a moment in your day to consciously pause, whether on your lunch break, at your desk or on your commute. Stop what you are doing and put down all electronics. (I know it's difficult!)

- *Notice:* Take three deep breaths. For at least five seconds, inhale. Then for five seconds, exhale. Notice what arises in the body and mind. What do you feel?

- *Catch:* Allow yourself to catch and place these emotions and thoughts in the palm of your hand as you extend your arm away from your body. View those sensations with an objective lens. How does it feel to acknowledge those emotions and thoughts as a separate entity and within your control?¬†

- *Release:* Take a couple deep breaths to simply be with those sensations without judgment. Then, put your hand to your mouth and blow those emotions away. Watch them dissipate into the air, leaving you to feel weightless and free.

- *Shift:* Recognize the shift in your energy as you free yourself and create space for the emotions you choose to feel. Smile and notice the positive vibrations tingle throughout your entire body.

- *Own:* Take ownership of your feelings and sensations.

Utilize them as indicators to better understanding your inner emotion code and what drives you. Feel inspired by your ability to boldly face and explore everything you feel without judgment.

***

This may feel a little out there if you've never explored how you feel, tried to understand the reasons for those feelings, or taken consistent action to change the way you feel. It certainly was new to me when I started changing my relationship landscape a decade ago.

Today, I work a lot with my clients on that matter. I help them think through their emotions and bring clarity in the decisions that need to be made. Discomfort and fear often come from feelings that are left unexplored. Speaking to someone, especially when you are disconnected from the mothership on the road, can help create a platform to explore your emotions and bring you peace.

EMMA'S STORY

During a Summer Gourmet Detox event I was leading, one of the participants, a woman in her 60s, could not sleep. I scheduled a private session with her and asked her what the matter was. She said: "I am sad and worried about my mother's health. She is dying and was relocated to a hospital two hours away. I'm scared to see her die and not have her around anymore, but there is nothing that I can do about it." Presented that way, the sleep issue looked unsolvable, until her mother passed.

I was not convinced that the root cause of my client's

suffering was her mother dying (call it power of intuition and years of putting myself in other people's shoes). I asked her if she wanted to talk things through a little more and get to the bottom of what was really nagging at her, the underlying feelings, so that she could make the decisions that would bring her peace. Without a clearer definition of the problem, there was no possible resolution.

After exploring her emotions for 10 minutes, the problem that emerged was redefined and became actionable. My client was not tortured because her mother was dying (however hard that is), but because she was not sitting by her side to enjoy her company while she was still alive.

The reason she could not be there was that she worked two jobs, across seven days a week, had no more vacation days and could not miss work, being a single mum paying college tuition for her two daughters. This was the real reason she felt stuck.

Quite a different perspective isn't it? Prompted by a few more questions, encouraged by a listening and non-judgmental ear, she was able to craft a solution that exposed her to new ways of working. She leveraged a professional network of 25 years that she had never tapped into in such a way. That very same night, she slept through the night, a huge weight off her shoulders and the next week she was by her mother's side.

This is how powerful it is to surround yourself with nurturing relationships and how digging into your emotions, especially uncomfortable ones, can lead to profound life transformation feeding your success.

Your turn!

Remember a time when your heart was heavy and how speaking about your worry made you feel better afterwards. What was asked? What was said? How did that conversation alleviate your worry? What did you do?

_____

_____

_____

_____

_____

_____

_____

_____

_____

_____

_____

_____

_____

_____

9
MILESTONE 5:
SLOW DOWN TO FOCUS AND
INNOVATE

Develop a relaxation and consciousness practice to reduce stress and slow down, to increase mental focus, self-reflection and stimulate your ability to visualize, think creatively and innovate.

The subject in this chapter may feel esoteric at first. It is both the most important and the most difficult milestone to achieve in GDN and it may require a lot of practice. That's because it is the holy grail for achieving a fulfilling and successful life. It did not even occur to me until I burned out and attended the Institute for Integrative Nutrition. There,

I studied with spiritual leaders like Deepak Chopra who taught me about consciousness and leadership as connected concepts and introduced me to meditation.

The reason slowing down is the holy grail of fulfillment is that there is no other time than now. The past is gone and the future never arrives. You always live in the present, in the now. Slowing down therefore improves your experience and enjoyment of the now. It enables you to focus all your power on what is going on right this second.

As your diet and lifestyle improve, you will start to feel a greater sense of calm and balance. Through this process, you will become more fully present in the moment.

By being more fully present, you have the opportunity to understand yourself more deeply because you have the time to hear the voice within, your intuition, with greater clarity. You can also feel your desires more strongly and understand what needs to be done now. Your actions become more impactful and you end up living the life you want to live. Your dreams of the future are the culmination of present moment after present moment, executed using your authentic self-expression. When you slow down, your focus and creativity are heightened, and subsequently feed your success.

This chapter introduces a few simple tools that can help you slow down.

Questions:

In an hour, how often do you think about the past?

_____

_____

And how often do you project yourself into or prepare something for the future?

_____

_____

How often and for how long are you able to focus on the present moment, right now?

_____

_____

What do you find the most challenging in trying to slow down?

_____

_____

_____

_____

_____

_____

Today's society is connected 24/7, without geographical or time boundaries, and with greater proximity to others through social media. This makes it virtually impossible to find 'me-time' or to dance to the beat of your own drum. The continuously fast-paced work schedule, with constant multi-tasking, sometimes to the point of oblivion and without any break makes the mere thought of attempting to slow down feel utterly rebellious. Exhaustion caused by long travel times, jetlag, overtime and being always 'on' reduces time allocated to sleep and keeps us feeling wired.

How on earth can we slow down? And where do we start?

To get going on this practice of slowing down, make sure you are operating under your new belief system. We lie to ourselves the most in relation to self-care. We come up with all sorts of excuses to justify why we cannot slow down, carve out some me-time, how taking care of ourselves is selfish, how we cannot ask for help unless we're in a crisis, that nothing will get done if we take time off, and that we are powerless.

If that is what's going on, revisit your beliefs. Understand where they're coming from. Challenge them. Ask yourself if you know them to be true. Then create new beliefs that support all the wonderful reasons you should carve out time for yourself and slow down.

Here is the list of prescriptions to help you slow down and improve your focus:

1	Develop a consciousness practice that works for you.
2	Practice the Relaxing Breath twice a day.
3	Use travel time as downtime.
4	Live mindfully.

Prescription 1: Develop a consciousness practice that works for you.

In today's fast-paced world, we all need to become more conscious and have a consciousness (or 'spiritual') practice. We all are spiritual beings in one sense or another. You included. You just need to find a practice that works for you. It's that bio-individuality thing again. Think about what you crave the most and build your consciousness practice around it.

EMMA'S STORY

> Living in concrete and populated New York, what I crave the most is nature and solitude. A walk in the park by myself or riding my road bike is what makes me feel most consciously focused, alive and rejuvenated.

A consciousness practice that works for you is one that fuels your mind and makes you feel connected with yourself, which in turn makes you feel good and happier. Think of it as a moment when you cherish yourself. It does not have to take a lot of time, or require complicated logistics. It is simply a special, sacred space for you.

A consciousness practice can take the form of prayer, meditation, a walk on the beach, chanting, dancing, yoga, journaling, free-writing the moment you wake up (also called morning pages), reading something spiritual, listening intently to music, and many more calming and tuned-in moments that you can imagine for yourself.

The right consciousness practice will uplift your soul, fill your heart with gratitude and love, make you feel magnificent, healthy and happy. *The most effective consciousness practice is the one you will practice daily.* Give yourself time to get good at it and use a timer to give your practice a beginning and an end, enabling you to fully focus and enjoy the experience.

Athletes are often spiritual, as it may help them cope with the challenges of competitions. One of the best books written on meditation (and which has been the bible to many American athletes) is *Thinking Body, Dancing Mind: Taosports for Extraordinary Performance in Athletics, Business, and Life* by Chungliang Al Huang and Jerry Lynch. I highly recommend it.

My consciousness practice could be:

_____

_____

_____

_____

The best moment of the day to set time for my practice could be:

_____

_____

_____

_____

In order to keep that time available and undisturbed (sacred), I need to:

_____

_____

_____

_____

Prescription 2: Practice the Relaxing Breath twice a day.

Another powerful way to slow down and focus on the moment (the starting point of another consciousness practice) is deep breathing. There are many types of breath and you can practice many techniques through Pranayama yoga. My favorite breathing technique is the 4-7-8 Relaxing Breath that I learned from Dr. Andrew Weil in nutrition school (Harvard graduate and founder, professor, and director of the Arizona Center for Integrative Medicine at the University of Arizona).

The Relaxing Breath has been linked to dramatic physiological health improvement, stress reduction and mental focus improvement. It helps me recharge and reconnect with myself and makes me feel a little high (all that oxygen!). It also leaves me feeling creative.

The Relaxing Breath Exercise

Sit up with your back straight. (Eventually you'll be able to do this in any position.) Put the tip of your tongue on the ridge behind your top front teeth; keep it there through the exercise.

- To begin, exhale through the mouth making a 'whoosh' sound.

- Close your mouth and inhale though your nose to the count of 4.

- Hold your breath for the count of 7.

- Exhale through your mouth, making a 'whoosh' sound for a count of 8.

- Repeat these steps four more times.

Do this exercise at least twice daily. You may repeat it more often, but don't do more than four breaths at a time.

Prescription 3: Use travel time as downtime.

Travelers, you're in luck! Your airplane (or train) commute can become your outlet to slow down, breathe, catch up on sleep, daydream, people-watch, do some undisturbed creative thinking, meditate, and read some inspirational writing. In other words, make the plane or train ride a spa trip and be determined to treat yourself in the best possible way during travel time.

After my meltdown episode, I boarded every plane with self-care in mind. For this reason, I cut back on red-eye flights. I would travel early morning, my most productive brain time. And I would fast during the flight, drink no alcohol, but make sure I had plenty of water and time to do all my self-care rituals: the Relaxing Breath, meditation, power napping, listening to classical music and reading inspirational books. On longer flights, I would add stretching and hours of creative thinking into the mix using an old-fashioned composition book. What is my next big idea? What are my clients' biggest pain points? What solutions do they wish I presented them? How do I develop the next generation of leaders in my team?

I used to use travel time to catch up on emails, work, report drafting and reviews, but realized that taking a break, when no-one expected an answer from me, was a much better use of my time.

Do not underestimate the power of taking a break and recovering. Athletes know that it is during recovery time that their bodies repair. The recovery is anabolic. It builds up the body. On the other hand, exercise is catabolic. It breaks down the body. It is not the exercise but the quality recovery from a training session that makes an athlete stronger. For the busy professional and business traveler, using travel time as down-time could be an easier way to unwind and rejuvenate.

Prescription 4: Live mindfully.

The last tip to help you slow down (and one which worked incredibly well for me) was to focus on living mindfully. Living mindfully means dedicating your full attention to what you are doing. This is extremely hard to do, but the ultimate goal, the holy grail, of living in the now.

To live mindfully:

- Stop multi-tasking. Do only one thing at a time and focus on that one task. However small and unimportant a task may seem, be it brushing your teeth, driving, or being on call, focus 100% on what it is you are doing.

- Eat mindfully. Eat without distraction. Put down the magazine. Turn off the TV, phone, computer. Sit in front of your plate at the kitchen or dinner table. Focus on your food, your surroundings, company, the presentation of your dish and enjoy the process of eating. This is such a calming practice. It increases satiety and reduces digestive stress, just like chewing...

- Chew your food thoroughly. Chewing begins the digestion process of carbohydrates by mixing digestive enzymes present in the saliva with the food. Proper chewing requires at least 30 to 50 chews per bite, until the food is completely liquefied. Have you ever chewed 30 times? Try it for one week at every meal. This will slow you down and enhance the pleasure of eating. You'll see.

- Take a minute at the beginning of the day to sit for a moment with your eyes closed when you start your computer.

- Reserve 15 minutes for yourself before starting your day to connect. Divide this time into 5-5-5. Take five minutes to do some journaling, another five minutes for reading something inspiring or listening to a song, and a final five minutes of silence and meditation.

- Let the phone ring a few times before picking it up or let it go to voicemail and listen to it when you finish the task you were engaged in.

- Take the scenic route to work.

- Create space in your calendar between appointments so that there's room for a short walk.

- Spend more time playing with your (or someone else's) kids. Children live in the now.

Write down three practices you'd like to try to live more mindfully:

_____
_____
_____
_____
_____
_____
_____
_____

EMMA'S STORY

It is by slowing down, practicing the exercises above, that I've been able to get more satisfaction and happiness out of my life, become more creative and see several stress symptoms dissipate (like memory loss).

The biggest surprise to me was that slowing down did not undermine the quality of my work in any way. It increased the pleasure I took in working, because I was really taking in all the multi-faceted experiences of my work and not feeling anxious or rushed anymore.

PART III
CALLING YOU INTO ACTION

Congratulations! You've learned so much, asked yourself many questions and already made some vital decisions about your health. The five milestones of goal-directed nutrition are interdependent. As you continue to improve upon them over the course of your life, you'll see a greater ripple effect on all the other milestones. And you'll become unstoppable!

To conclude, I want to leave you with a few thoughts about the best way to implement GDN.

Follow the sequence of the five milestones, as they build on each other, everything of course starting with the food:

- Start with adding the good food; that is the most nutrient-dense foods and drink the right amount of water. Crowd out the harmful foods. Get organized, try to cook as much as possible. And when dining out, stick with the rules no matter what.

- As you start to feel better because of the food intake, turn your attention to improving your sleep. There again, you'll need to make decisions to reorganize your life around your sleep schedule. Create a ritual you can consistently apply, day after day, and communicate your priority for getting some good quality sleep to the people in your life. Ask for their support.

- As you bring the food and sleep under control, your body will be in greater shape to handle a new exercise routine. If you are beginner, invest in a trainer to learn the basics of good form, to avoid contra-indicated movements and to pace yourself adequately. Alternatively, you could join group fitness classes. Start super-slow and focus on being consistent, doing something every day, scheduling exercise in your calendar. Exercise is about establishing a new healthy lifestyle. Remember that exercise as short as 10 minutes daily can be the right place to start.

- Soon your body will feel so good, your mind so clear, that you'll experience a deep sense of balance. This is the right foundation to begin exploring your feelings and emotions, and revamp your relationships landscape to meet your needs. Tackling emotions and building relationships earlier in the process, when you eat junk food that clouds your mind and makes you feel chronically exhausted and uncomfortable in your body, is hardly the right place to start.

- Finally, the holy grail of feeding success is to be able to slow down and be fully in the present moment. Only in the present moment, can you leave your mark and make an impact. If you learn how to concentrate and master all your talents, and use your formidable health, intuition and perception to guide their application, you'll be unbeatable.

I cannot wait to see what you're capable of. The world needs you to play big so go get started. Best of luck!

APPENDIX 1: On-The-Go Snacks

All these snacks are real wholesome foods.

Travel with bottled water. Drink often to differentiate a craving for food from dehydration.

Salty Snacks	Crunchy
Seasnax, spicy nori strips (seaweed)	Organic apples and pears
Olives	Carrots
Sauerkraut and vegetables pickles	Celery and real peanut butter
Hummus, tabouli	Mocchi
Edamame	Rice cakes with almond butter
Kale chips	Plain popcorn
Steamed or raw vegetables with tamari/shoyu or umeboshi vinegar	Dehydrated vegetables chips
	Unsalted and untoasted nuts and seeds
Creamy	**Sweet**
Guacamole, avocado dip with veggies	Fresh fruit, berries
Hummus and baba ganoush dips	Dates stuffed with nut butter
Creamy soup	Dried fruit (apricot, figs, mango, raisins)
Rice pudding	
Mashed sweet potato	Smoothies
Coconut milk, almond milk, coconut yogurt, kefir	Baked sweet vegetables (squashes, sweet potatoes) sprinkled with cinnamon
Full fat yogurt from grass-fed cow	Oat drink or porridge with fruit, maple syrup, cinnamon, cardamom, vanilla bean and nut milk
Frozen banana pureed with cinnamon	

APPENDIX 2: Feeding Success Superfoods Trail Mix

Organic Ingredients: sunflower seeds, pumpkin seeds, cashews, coconut flakes, raw cacao nibs, goji berries and dark raisins.

Cacao (superfood): Rich mineral content, #1 source of magnesium, the highest concentration of antioxidants of any food in the world, feel-good effect from phenylethylamine (PEA). Together, PEA and magnesium are great appetite suppressants.

Coconut (superfood): Fast energy from the medium chain fatty acids; hormonal, immune and nervous system support; belly fat burning effect; antiviral, antibacterial and antifungal properties.

Goji berries (superfood): Most nutritionally dense berry on the planet, only food source known to stimulate production of human growth hormone, an adaptogen with many therapeutic effects. Complete protein.

Sunflower seeds: Very high in vitamin E (heart health) and selenium (anti-cancer), helps lower LDL cholesterol. The antidote seed for a stressful life!

Pumpkin seeds: Antidepressant, lowering LDL cholesterol, mineral and vitamins dense, treat prostate and bladder problems.

Raisins: Most alkaline food on earth!

Cashews: Anti-depressant, anti-anxiety, well-being and 'no worries' effect stemming from high levels of l-triptophan.

APPENDIX 3: Feeding Success 4-Day Menu Sample 1 (Late Summer)

Go to blog.zenberrymix.com where all recipes and more meal plans with flavors of the world are available for download.

All the recipes below are compliant with the GDN diet and 100% homemade in less than 15 minutes.

	Monday	**Tuesday**	**Wednesday**	**Thursday**
Breakfast	Collard Greens w/ Mango Smoothie	Spinach w/Apple Smoothie	Collard Greens w/Mango Smoothie	Spinach w/Apple Smoothie
Lunch	Spiced Cauliflower w/Sesame Seeds	Chickpea & Summer Squash Salad	Collard Rolls w/Hummus + Summer Squash Soup	Collard Greens Topped w/ Tomato & Chickpea Curry
Snack	Melon w/ Mint	Hummus w/Veggies	Melon w/Mint	Hummus w/ Veggies
Dinner	Tomato & Chickpea Curry	Spiced Cauliflower w/Sesame Seeds + Sweet Corn & Collard Green Sauté	Chickpea Corn Salad	Cauliflower Tomato Herb Stuffed Summer Squash
Dessert	Banana Cinnamon Ice Cream	Chia Seed Pudding w/ Mango & Blueberries	Banana Cinnamon Ice Cream	Chia Seed Pudding w/ Mango & Blueberries

APPENDIX 4: Feeding Success 4-Day Menu Sample 2 (On The Road)

Go to blog.zenberrymix.com where all recipes are available for download.

Monday	Tuesday	Wednesday	Thursday
1 glass of water + Alkaline Booster (Orange or Grapefruit Juice with Spirulina)			
Overnight oats with chia seeds and raisins	1 cup oatmeal + berries + chia seeds	1 cup fruit salad: pineapple and watermelon or berries	2 whole (organic) eggs omelet with 1 cup spinach, 1 tomato, onions, red peppers and black pepper
Caesar Salad or Chicken on Greens	**Colorful Salad** (vegetarian) Leafy greens, red, yellow, purple, white vegetables, seeds or nuts, ½ an avocado and 1 cup legumes (chickpeas or beans), a splash of lemon and olive oil and vinegar dressing.	**Cruciferous Vegetables Salad** (vegan) Include cauliflower, or broccoli, or kale, or cabbage in your salad.	**Quinoa Salad** (vegan) Quinoa with raw and cooked vegetables and healthy fats like avocado, seeds or nuts.
Early night rest at the hotel. A vegetarian soup and a couple of side vegetable dishes. No alcohol.	**Mediterranean Team Dinner.** Wild salmon, trout or branzini with vegetables. Max 1 drink.	**Steak House Client Dinner.** 3 oz grass-fed steak (share), 2 sides of leafy greens. Max 1 drink.	**Airport Meal.** Japanese veggie and avocado roll, seaweed salad, or hummus and veggie platter.

APPENDIX 5: Feeding Success Power Breakfasts

Overnight Superfoods Oats	Super-Immunity Shake	Power Fruit Salad
Ingredients:	**Ingredients:**	**Ingredients:**
1/3 cup of raw oats	8 to 10 oz coconut water (with flesh if using fresh coconut)	1/2 a ripe avocado
1 tsp of raw honey	1 cup spinach	1 cup papaya
1 tsp of cinnamon	1/2 banana	2 fresh figs
1 tsp of cardamom	1 inch cube of raw beet peeled	1 tbsp cinnamon
½ cup of coconut nut milk	1/4 cup frozen blueberries	2 tbsp of lemon juice (or more)
1 tbsp of goji berries	**Superfoods boosters:**	1 peach with the skin or 1 nectarine
1 tbsp of chia seeds and hemp seeds	1 tbsp chia seeds	1 tbsp raw honey
1 tbsp raw cacao nibs	1 tbsp bee pollen (or raw honey)	1 pinch of Himalayan pink salt (optional for additional minerals)
1 tbsp coconut oil	1 tbsp raw cacao nibs	1 pinch of cayenne pepper
1 tsp algae powder (spirulina or chlorella)	**Directions:** Begin mixing the liquid with the beet, and frozen berries. Add the banana, spinach and the boosters last. Bon appétit!	**Directions:** Mix the honey, lemon juice, cayenne pepper and pink salt and let the dressing rest while you chop all the fruit and present them nicely. Pour the dressing on the fruit, and sprinkle the cinnamon over. Voilà!
1 pinch of Himalayan pink salt		
Directions: Mix everything in a mason jar and let it soak overnight. It is ready to savor in the morning and easily transported in the mason jar to work.		

APPENDIX 6: Dining-Out Questionnaire

Does your restaurant have filtered tap water?
Are there any raw or cooked leafy greens on the menu?
Are there any other vegetable dishes (tomatoes, cauliflower, broccoli, asparagus, sweet potatoes, Brussels sprouts, root vegetables, corn on the cob, and other whole grains)?   (If there is a choice, choose organic, non-GMO vegetables.)
Where does the meat and chicken come from and how was it raised?   (Is the beef pastured and grass-fed? Is the chicken free-roaming organic-fed?)
Is the salmon wild-caught? What other fish do you have? Where does it come from? Is it farm-raised or wild-caught?
How is it cooked? May I have it broiled, steamed, water sautéed, baked? If prepared with fat, can you only use butter or olive oil?   (Ensure no vegetable shortening.)
May I have the dressing or the sauce served separately on the side?
May I substitute items like French fries or macaroni and cheese for green vegetables, baked sweet potato or boiled potatoes, even if it costs more?
May I order something special? Could the chef make me a vegetarian beans and vegetables dish, even though it's not on the menu?
May I order a main course size of the salad appetizer or vegetable side dish?
Could you keep away the bread and serve this dish without [bacon, fries, sausage, and any other ingredients you may be tempted to eat if put in front of you]?

Appendix 7: Sample On-The-Go Workout Schedule*

	Morning	Lunch/ During the Day	Evening
Monday (Early Travel)	10 Sun Salutations OR 3 sets of push-ups & 3 sets of sit-ups to exhaustion – It takes 10 minutes!	15 min. walk after lunch	Run before dinner for 20 to 30 min. (after dropping suitcase at the hotel) or/and long digestive walk after dinner
Tuesday	An indoor cycling or bootcamp class at the local gym or an Action DVD or Bliss Yoga DVD	15 min. walk after lunch	A gentle yoga or pilates in my bedroom (Candlelit Yoga or Pilates DVD by Crunch Fitness or self-created routine)
Wednes-day	Weight lifting or circuit training for 30 to 45 min at the hotel gym: 1 min per exercise, alternating upper body with lower body exercises and integrating balance training in the routine (unstable surfaces or 1 leg up)	15 min. walk after lunch	Core training for 20 min. in my room before showering or taking a bath focusing on abdominals (obliques, transversal rotations, planks, crunches, scissors, etc.), back (extension, rotation, flexion), gluteus and hips (extension, abduction, adduction, flexion). An exercise a minute moving in all planes of motion, standing and laying down, without rest.

Thursday (Late Travel)	Swimming in the hotel pool for 20 minutescontinuously, or an interval class at the local gym or an intense interval run (or walk / sprint intervals).	15 min. walk after lunch	Walk the airport terminal for 30 minutes and get a back rub at the "Express Spa" if time allows.

I travel with 1 action and 1 relaxing DVD, a Yamuna ball to stretch using myofascial release almost daily as well as resistance bands sometimes. I also always have my workout playlists to motivate me.

* Please consult with a physician before engaging in any exercise regimen.

ABOUT THE AUTHOR

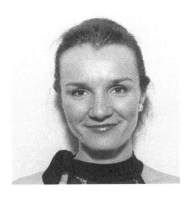

Emmanuelle was born and raised in France. She attended college in France and later, Sweden, where she lived for 6 years. Shortly after graduating, Emma landed a job with one of the "Big Four" professional services firms in Malmö, Sweden, starting her fast-paced and challenging corporate career. After living and working in Switzerland for 3 years, Emma moved to the US where her love for fitness and nutrition blossomed. She holds certifications in personal training, group fitness, Spinning, and many others. Emma is also a certified holistic health and nutrition coach through The Institute of Integrated Nutrition and the American Association of Drugless Practitioners. From her practice based in NYC, she helps clients throughout the world transform their life, using health as a catalyst.

Stay Connected with Emmanuelle

If you want to get an automatic email when Emma releases Feeding Success meal plans and nutrition and lifestyle tips for the busy professional and business travelers, sign up for her free goji fitness newsletter at www.gojifitness.com

Help Emmanuelle out

Word-of-mouth is crucial for any author to succeed. If you enjoyed the book, please consider leaving a review where you purchased it, even if it is only a line or two; it would make all the difference and would be very much appreciated.

Meet Emmanuelle

If you're interested in having Emmanuelle speak at your organization or want to set up a Feeding Success challenge for your team, contact her at emma@gojifitness.com

In all of Emmanuelle's presentations, you will discover new food and take part in gentle exercise or stretching to leave you energized, inspired and better connected with others.